Freedom

Freedom
The Smart Parents Guide How to Help Your Child See a Better Life

Dr. Mark J. Page, OD
with

Dr. David Roth, OD, Dr. Stuart Grant, OD

Dr. Dale Tosland, OD, Dr. David Bartels, OD

Dr. Michael Murphy, OD

Dr. Kevin Reeder, OD, Dr. Earl Sandler, OD

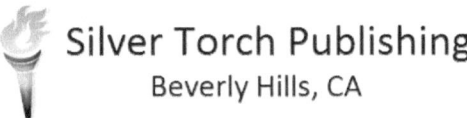

Silver Torch Publishing
Beverly Hills, CA

Freedom: The Smart Parents Guide How to Help Your Child See a Better Life
©2016 by Dr. Mark J. Page, O.D.

www.thesmartparentsguide.com

Cover design by Katie Benedikt.

Printed in the United States of America.

Paperback ISBN: 978-1-942707-49-3
LCCN: 2017934499

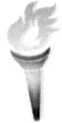
Published by Silver Torch Press
www.SilverTorchPress.com
Jill@SilverTorchPress.com

All rights reserved. No part of this book may be reproduced or transmitted in any form or by any means without written permission from the author.

Information provided in this book is for informational purposes only. This information is NOT intended as a substitute for the advice provided by your physician or other healthcare professional, or any information contained on or in any product.

Do not use the information provided in this book for diagnosing or treating a health problem or disease, or prescribing medication or other treatment. Always speak with your physician or other healthcare professional before taking any medication or nutritional, herbal or homeopathic supplement, or using any treatment for a health problem. If you have or suspect that you have a medical problem, contact your health care provider promptly. Do not disregard professional medical advice or delay in seeking professional advice because of something you have read in this book.

Dedication

This book is dedicated to all of the amazing patients and parents with whom we work with on a daily basis. Our wish for this book is to help educate parents and potential patients about the risk factors and warning signs of eye disease, and what you can do to potentially reduce the risks of myopia. Our lives revolve around our eyesight. We are excited to provide this information about the benefits of orthokeratology to help you and your child see a better life.

Contents

Chapter 1: The Myopia Epidemic 1

Chapter 2: Eye Diseases and Reducing Your Risk 13

Chapter 3: How Myopia Can Lead to Retinal Detachment 24

Chapter 4: Corrective Eye Surgery 29

Chapter 5: Major Risk Factors for Developing Myopia 39

Chapter 6: A Case for Myopia Control Now 47

Chapter 7: Options for Myopia Control 53

Chapter 8: The Gold Standard 61

Chapter 9: Orthokeratology Stuart Grant, O.D. 66

Chapter 10: Who Benefits From Ortho-K? 75

Chapter 11: The Benefits of Ortho-K for Children 86

Chapter 12: The Benefits of Ortho-K for Adults 97

Chapter 13: What to Expect When Getting Ortho-K Aligners 107

Chapter 14: Choosing a Doctor for Ortho-K 112

Chapter 15: Here's to Your Eye Health! 121

Acknowledgments

I would like to acknowledge my publisher Jill Fagan and her husband David, who gave me the faith that this book could be done. I also would like to acknowledge Dr. Nick Despotidis, who shared with me that writing a book was one of the best things he ever did. To my associates Dr. Alma Yamamoto and Dr. Kurt Jung who are always there to keep the ship moving forward. My entire staff including Sandy and Joe Szymczak and my wife Gina, who believe in me and encourage me to conquer this amazing project.

CHAPTER ONE

The Myopia Epidemic

The number of people with poor vision, blindness, eye diseases, and the need for glasses and contacts is skyrocketing at an alarming rate, not just in our country, but all over the world. According to *Research America*, "the population of people with vision loss and blindness is estimated to increase by approximately 150 percent" by the year 2050. This rate of increase means deteriorating eye health is becoming a worldwide epidemic, and at an annual cost of about $145 billion, the burden isn't exclusive to those with poor vision. That is an "estimated cost of $6,680 per person per year," with approximately 48 percent of those costs being paid through government funding and health insurance—in other words, your taxes and health care premiums (*Research America*).

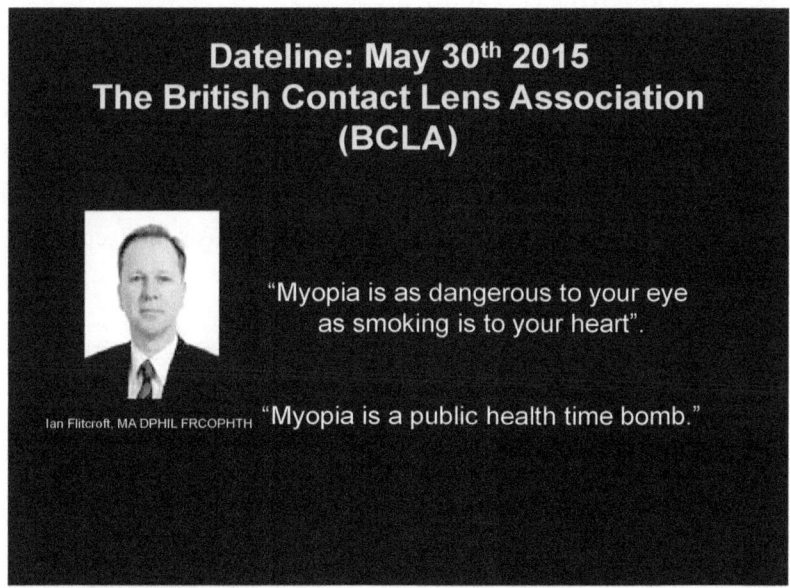

However, there isn't just the financial cost that comes with this rising epidemic, but an emotional one as well. Just imagine how much your life would change if you or your loved one developed an eye disease or became blind. Would you still be able to work or do the things you enjoy? Would you be able to care for yourself, or would a family member need to care for you? The point is that poor vision can dramatically reduce your quality of life.

Today, vision problems are so common that we hardly notice those who wear glasses anymore. Just a few decades ago, glasses seemed reserved for the bookish or elderly, yet now they have become mainstream. The eye-care industry has greatly expanded the options and styles available, making them more like accessories. Likewise, contact lens companies have expanded their options to ensure that more people can wear contacts, even if they don't need correction to their vision. Consumers can purchase contacts to change the look and color of their eyes. Contact lens companies have also moved away from hard contacts, promoting disposable soft lenses as more comfortable and feasible for more people. They have introduced a wide variety of lenses, each designed to best suit patients' varied needs.

The corrective lens industry generates billions of dollars a year, and that doesn't include the amount spent on LASIK and other laser eye surgeries. "Eye disorders are the fifth most expensive chronic condition to treat" (*Research America*). Children currently make up about 4 percent of the eye care costs in this country. This may not seem like much, but the number of children developing vision problems is steadily increasing.

So, why are children needing glasses at younger and younger ages? Some may argue that it is simply because we now have the technology to better detect poor eyesight. However, research shows that the prevalence of poor eyesight is clearly on the rise both in the United States, as well as in many foreign countries. Experts are predicting poor eyesight to become a catastrophic health concern, creating unprecedented suffering and astronomical costs that could bankrupt our health-care system. Yet, the general public remains mostly unaware of this potentially devastating epidemic.

The high cost of high myopia

- **The medical burden of high myopia includes pathologic complications such as myopic macular degeneration, choroidal neovascularisation, cataract and glaucoma.[1]**
- **Uncorrected refractive error could also impair vision-related quality of life and increase difficulty in performing vision-related tasks.[4]**

While some vision problems are treatable, most can cause vision loss that is often permanent. Our focus needs to be not on treating vision problems as they occur, when it is typically too late to reverse the damage, but on preventing them. This is why it is so important to reduce the prevalence of vision problems in children now. By protecting our children's eyesight, we will effectively reduce the estimated rise in vision loss in the future, and reduce the financial and emotional costs that go along with vision loss.

There are five common vision problems a child may experience. The first is amblyopia, or lazy eye. This is when one eye does not connect properly with the brain. The vision in that eye is usually worse than that of the other eye, even when the child wears glasses. If left untreated, lazy eye can cause long-term vision loss.

The second eye condition common among children is astigmatism. This is caused by the cornea being irregularly shaped. Astigmatism

Madeline and Daniel are my kids. As both their father and doctor, I'm happy my children's myopic progression stopped once they started molding. My wife is a -5.00 D. Thankfully the kids are still -1.00 OU after 13 years of molding."

David P. Bartels OD

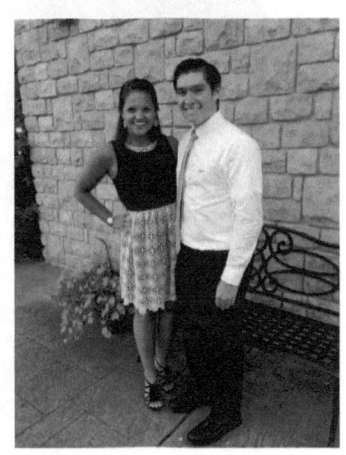

can negatively impact both close-range and long-distance vision. It is generally something an individual is born with, and having a family history of astigmatism greatly increases the risk.

The third common vision problem in children is strabismus, which is when the two eyes are not working together. This can result in a wandering eye, the eyes being turned in or turned out. Strabismus can cause amblyopia—poor vision with no apparent defects to the eyes themselves—double vision or vision in only one eye.

Hyperopia, or farsightedness, is the fourth vision problem common among children. This is when the individual can see objects at far distances clearly but struggles with things that are at close range. Some small children with hyperopia outgrow this condition as their eyes develop more fully.

The fifth and most common vision problem in children, and the focus of this book, is myopia. As known as nearsightedness, myopia is when the individual can see clearly at close distances but has trouble focusing on objects that are farther away. Myopia is estimated to become the most common vision problem in children. Myopia can be progressive, so people with the condition typically experience a worsening of their vision over time. Myopia is also a significant contributing factor to several serious eye diseases and conditions, such as retinal detachment, glaucoma, and cataracts, all of which can result in permanent vision loss. The more severe the nearsightedness, the higher the risk for developing a potentially blinding eye condition.

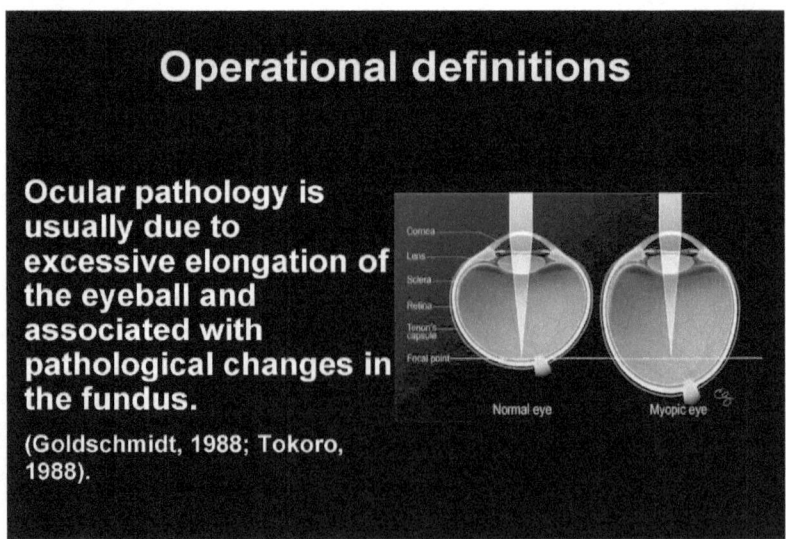

Myopia can be hereditary, but most commonly, it develops over time as the eyeball elongates. When the eye stretches, the light entering the eye is no longer focused properly on the retina. Think of your eyes like a camera. The cornea, the clear front cover of the eyeball, and the human lens, act like the lens of a camera by focusing the light that enters the eye. The retina is like the film in a camera. It covers the inside of the back of the eyeball and *captures* the light focused on it to create the images we see.

As myopia progresses, the retina can stretch. This is referred to as elongation. The more the retina stretches, the more light is focused in front of the retina instead of directly on it. This makes it difficult to clearly see things farther away. As myopia progresses, the distance at which you can see things clearly decreases. When the retina stretches, the eye is actually getting longer, which puts strain on everything else in the eye, including the macula and the optic nerve. Myopia can be progressive, so once the retina starts elongating, it tends to continue doing so.

In addition to heredity, another common cause for myopia is visual stress, which can result from too much close work. However, there are other causes, such as health conditions like diabetes, which can negatively impact your vision.

Myopia is typically diagnosed through a vision test which uses the Snellen Eye Chart. The chart displays a series of letters that get progressively smaller as you work your way down. Once myopia is diagnosed, most eye doctors prescribe corrective lenses designed to fix the refractive errors and provide clear vision. The prescription of the lenses represents the difference between the patient's vision and perfect vision. The poorer the patient's vision is, the stronger his or her prescription will be.

Many schools start doing vision tests with kindergarteners and first graders. However, there are common signs parents can watch for that may indicate their child has a vision problem. These common signs include:

- Constantly squinting
- Holding books or other reading material extremely close to their faces
- Tilting their heads to one side when focusing on something
- Sitting too close to the television, computer, or tablet
- Easily losing their places while reading
- Covering one eye while reading or watching television
- Tracking with their finger while reading
- Light sensitivity
- Frequent headaches
- Constantly rubbing their eyes

While myopia is not a new problem by any means, it is clear that the prevalence of myopia is dramatically increasing in many parts of the world, raising it to epidemic status. Research conducted to gain a better understanding of why there has been such a rise in myopia indicates that many environmental and lifestyle factors play a significant role. These include our increased time spent on near work such as reading, watching television, using electronic devices, or doing detailed crafts like sewing. The lack of sunshine and reduced time spent outside, which often coincides with near work, also play a huge role. Our eyes are not designed to be constantly focused on close-up objects. Staying inside not only stops the eyes from being able to focus at great distances, but it also deprives us of the benefits of natural sunlight. Studies are also being conducted on what experts are calling Peripheral Retinal Defocus Theory. The theory is that the use of glasses and soft contacts also contributes to the progression of myopia.

The prevalence of myopia has increased significantly in developed regions such as the United States and Western Europe, but the greatest increase has been identified in Asian countries, most notably China. One study to explain this increase was conducted in southern China. A population-based, multi-generational study, it looked at the increase in myopia prevalence from one generation to the next. One group examined as part of this study consisted of fifteen-year-olds, while the second group was made up of their parents. This study found that the prevalence of myopia in the parents was 19.8 percent, yet in the children, it was 78.4 percent. This is clearly a significant jump from one generation to the next.

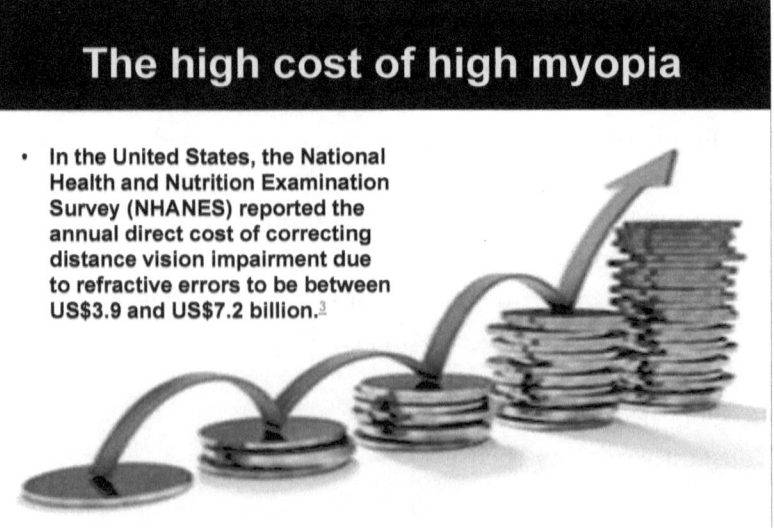

The high cost of high myopia

- In the United States, the National Health and Nutrition Examination Survey (NHANES) reported the annual direct cost of correcting distance vision impairment due to refractive errors to be between US$3.9 and US$7.2 billion.[3]

Other studies conducted in East Asia found that myopia among high school graduates was as high as 80 to 90 percent. According to *nature.com*, "In Seoul, a whopping 96.5 percent of nineteen-year-old men are short-sighted." With nearly all high school graduates dealing with poor vision, needing corrective lenses or corrective surgery, they are also all dealing with the increased risks associated with long-term myopia. That means 80 to 90 percent of the population in East Asia will be at a significant risk for eye diseases and retinal detachment as they age. With those increased risks come the increased financial and emotional costs associated with poor eyesight and blindness.

The National Health and Nutrition Examination Survey determined the prevalence of myopia in the United States between 1971 and 1972 was 25 percent. However, that same survey reported that between 1999 and 2004, the prevalence of myopia was 41.6 percent. That is a 66 percent increase in fewer than thirty years. The prevalence of myopia also affects all demographic groups. It is a cross-cultural issue as it is not associated with race, ethnicity, gender, or social-economic status.

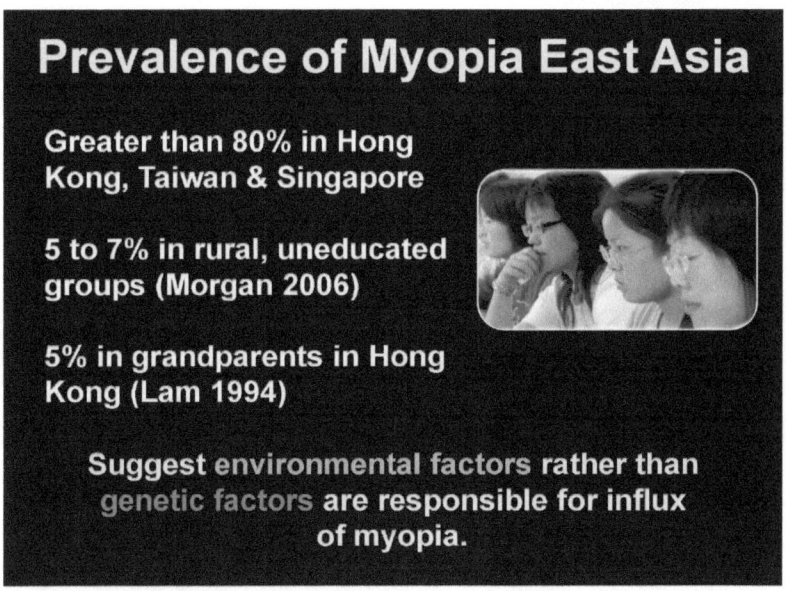

Prevalence of Myopia East Asia

Greater than 80% in Hong Kong, Taiwan & Singapore

5 to 7% in rural, uneducated groups (Morgan 2006)

5% in grandparents in Hong Kong (Lam 1994)

Suggest environmental factors rather than genetic factors are responsible for influx of myopia.

A study in Singapore found that the prevalence of myopia in the 1970s was at 26 percent. That increased to 43 percent by the late 1980s, 66 percent by the mid-1990s, and 80 percent by the late 1990s. The research proved that the increase in prevalence of myopia in Singapore has not only increased significantly, but it has increased quickly. The increase has been so dramatic that Singapore has turned to a public health approach to deal with the situation, since it is such a widespread problem.

Myopia is most prevalent in countries where children often watch television, play video games, or are otherwise engaged with electronic devices instead of playing outside. Recent research has shown that in large Asian cities such as Tokyo and Hong Kong, 30 to 50 percent of twelve-year-olds are already showing signs of myopia. Comparatively, in the United States, approximately 20 percent of twelve-year-olds show signs of myopia.

A study conducted on first-year college students in the United Kingdom found that 50 percent of them were myopic. In Greece, a study of fifteen to eighteen-year-olds showed that 36.8 percent had already developed the condition. Another study examining Western Europeans over the age of forty found that approximately 50 percent were myopic.

These statistics are surprising, but when compared to countries that are still developing, where most children don't have access to television or other electronics, the numbers become even more significant. In India, the prevalence of myopia is only 6.9 percent. Populated areas of Brazil are at 6.4 percent, and in Northwestern Brazil, which is populated mostly by indigenous people, the prevalence is only 2.7 percent. These statistics support the impact that close work and lack of sunshine have on the eyes.

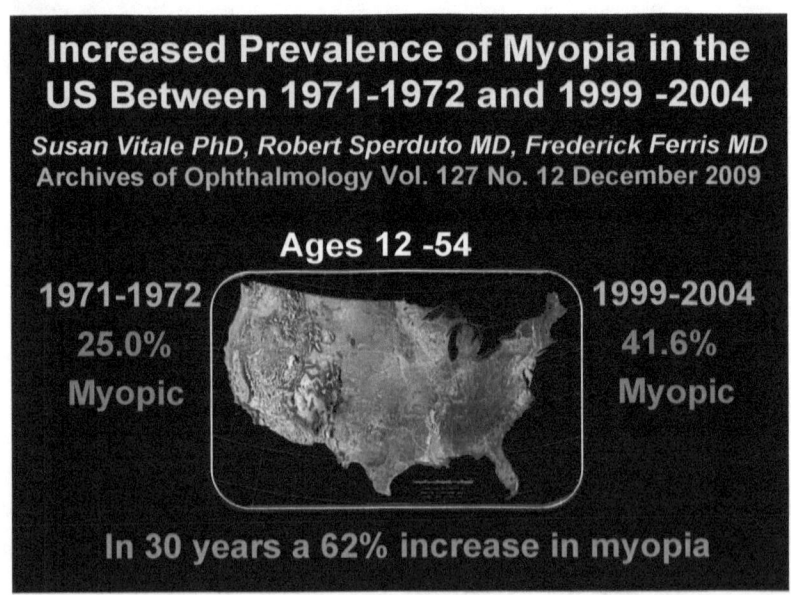

While myopia is a serious eye condition that should not be taken lightly, there are things you can do to protect yours and your child's eyesight. One of the ways you can control myopia is to simply spend more time outside. The human eye was not designed to focus on objects mere inches or feet away in low light. It was designed to see long distances in natural sunlight, and that can only be truly accomplished outside. Your eyes should be allowed to regularly focus on objects that are more than twenty feet away from you.

Not only do children spend a good portion of their day inside a classroom, many of them, as young as kindergarten, are now doing their school work on tablets and computers. This makes it nearly impossible for them to avoid the use of electronic devices. However, there are steps parents and teachers can take to help decrease the potential damage to children's eyesight.

Traditionally, the use of glasses has been associated with *smart kids*. While that is no longer the case, spending a great deal of time reading and studying does increase the risk of myopia significantly. In 2008, there was a study that reviewed the connection between myopia and IQ, as well as myopia and school achievement across several different countries. There are several proposed explanations for this connection. The first explanation is that studious children read and study more than the average, and it is this extra time spent on near work that causes their myopia. Among people with twelve or more years of formal education, the prevalence of myopia is as high as 59.8 percent. However, some have suggested that myopic children are better adapted to reading and test-taking, which impacts their performance on tests including the IQ test. While the connections have been supported across multiple studies, the exact cause has not been determined.

Several studies conducted primarily in Asian countries have also looked at the connection between education level and myopia. These studies have shown that the degree of myopia increases with the student's academic level. This connection is attributed to multiple factors including the amount of time spent doing near work, school achievement, time spent reading for pleasure, and language ability. These results were further supported by studies conducted in Asia, which demonstrated the progressively increasing prevalence of myopia by grade level.

Although there are many who still attribute the development of myopia primarily to hereditary factors, the heredity argument cannot explain the increase in prevalence over the last forty years. Myopia prevalence was relatively stagnant for many years, but since the 1970s, the percentage of myopic individuals has steadily increased. Myopia is also developing in children of younger and younger ages and at greater severity.

The increased prevalence of myopia in developed countries is clearly a fast-growing problem. However, why the sudden need for it to be treated as a public health concern? Why should parents be urged to consider myopia-control measures instead of settling for traditional corrective lenses? One reason would be that approximately $12 billion dollars a year is spent on corrective lenses in the United States alone.

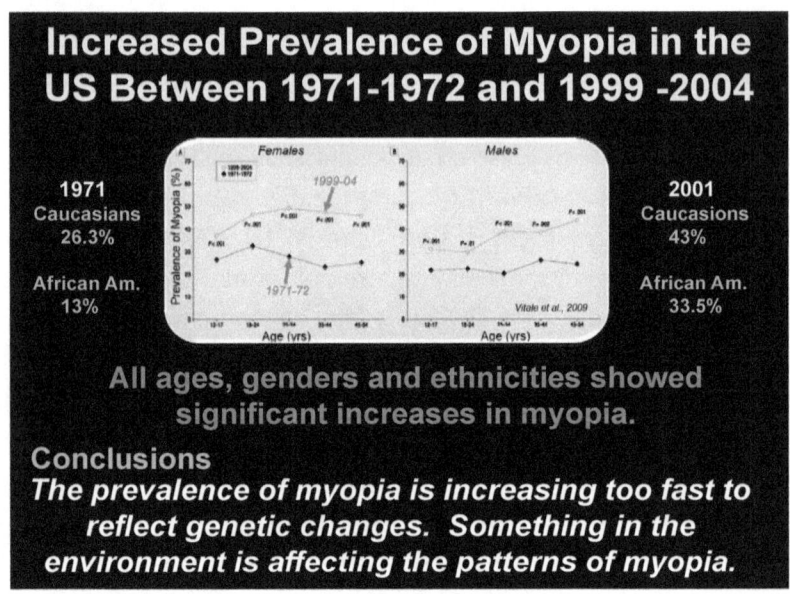

Research has also found that wearing corrective lenses, whether glasses or contacts, can increase the severity of the myopia over time. This is due to peripheral retinal defocus theory, which will be discussed in greater detail in a later chapter. Other complications can come from traditional methods of correction as well. For example, wearing contacts can increase the chances of developing an eye infection.

The risks associated with myopia are significant and can cause permanent vision loss. With the dramatic increase in young people developing myopia, there will be a significant rise in older adults with severe eye problems in the coming years. As explained earlier, myopia increases due to corneal elongation. Long-term and severe myopia have been associated with the development of cataracts, glaucoma, macular degeneration, peripheral retinal changes, along with retinal detachment, holes, and tears. These eye diseases and conditions can cause permanent eye damage or blindness.

Most of the possible treatments for these conditions involve surgery, which adds more risk to the overall situation. Furthermore, once vision loss has occurred, it cannot be restored. For example, if an individual developed glaucoma, treatment can prevent the further deterioration of their vision, but any vision that has already been lost cannot be recovered. Cataracts can be removed, or corneas transplanted, which may restore some vision. However, these eye surgeries can also increases the risk of retinal detachment.

Over recent years, LASIK eye surgery has become a popular means of correcting myopia. However, the general public's understanding of LASIK is often incorrect. Since LASIK uses a laser to reshape the cornea, it only corrects current nearsightedness. It does not stop the progression of myopia as it does not affect the retina nor stop it from stretching. It is important to understand that should your myopia continue to progress, you may need to go back to wearing glasses within just a few years following LASIK surgery. Corrective eye surgeries can also cause corneal scarring, itching, redness, dryness, and blurred vision among other complications. In rare cases, patients experience vision loss due to the corrective surgery.

Traditional correction methods only provide a temporary fix for the underlying problem. Controlling myopia is the only way to truly treat this condition, and for children, it is more important now than ever before. Once you have an understanding of the risks associated with long-term and severe myopia, the dangers of being diagnosed with myopia at a young age become clear. Still, it is never too late to take control of nearsightedness.

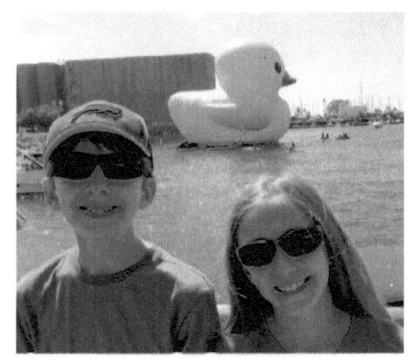

"Corneal molds are great for sports, swimming, and camping. I like them because I don't have to worry about any glasses falling off, and I don't have to worry about breaking them."

~ Jacob Murphy, 12

'Braces for the eyes'

There is an option, and that option is orthokeratology, which some call braces for the eyes. This book is a collaboration of some of the leading providers of orthokeratology who will examine the many options for myopia control in greater detail later in this book. These methods have been proven through research and been used successfully for many years. However, it is important to first understand the dangers of not getting myopia under control, especially in young children. If left to progress, myopia can lead to serious eye diseases and conditions that could mean blindness for you or your child later in life.

We will examine the many options for myopia control in greater detail later in this book. These methods have been proven through research and been used successfully for many years. However, it is important to first understand the dangers of not getting myopia under control, especially in young children. If left to progress, myopia can lead to serious eye diseases and conditions that could mean blindness for you or your child later in life.

CHAPTER TWO

Eye Diseases and Reducing Your Risk

Severe myopia is now believed to be a contributing risk factor for the development of multiple eye diseases, most notably glaucoma, cataracts, and macular degeneration. Researchers are also finding that the visual stress caused by the elongation of the eyeball can lead to retinal detachments and situations where eye diseases may develop more readily. As mentioned in the previous chapter, both glaucoma and macular degeneration are only treatable to a degree, and any vision loss that occurs is irreversible. Although the vision loss associated with cataracts is treatable, it is only treatable through surgery. However, studies suggest that cataract surgery can actually increase the risk of retinal detachment.

The older you get, and the more severe your myopia, the more likely you are to start developing any of these devastating eye diseases. Because of the projected increase in the prevalence of myopia in children, controlling their myopia now may dramatically decrease their risk of developing these diseases as they age. However, the benefits of controlling myopia aren't just for children. These eye diseases develop most commonly in patients over the age of fifty. Even if you are already at an increased risk for eye diseases, controlling your myopia may reduce your chances of developing them.

However, controlling myopia does not entirely eliminate your risk of developing these eye diseases. Heredity plays a role. If you have a family member who has been diagnosed with an eye disease, your chances of developing the same disease might be higher than someone with no family history. Your eyes will also continue to degenerate as you age, which can make a significant difference in your level of risk. By taking measures to get your myopia under control now, you will not only be reducing your risk, but you will be more likely to notice any changes to your vision sooner. As with any disease, early detection is key and can reduce your chances of permanent vision loss. Since most eye diseases are painless, noticing any kind of change in your vision should be cause to see your eye doctor.

Because there are other risk factors associated with the development of eye diseases, it is important to understand the symptoms and to get regular eye exams, especially if you have a family history of eye disease. Each of these conditions are treatable to some extent. However, the earlier they are detected, the more options you will have when facing treatment.

Our vision affects so many areas of our lives, and although a loss of vision isn't fatal, it will dramatically impact your quality of life—your ability to work, pursue hobbies or further education. Controlling myopia should truly be treated as a public health concern. Just as children are taught that avoiding tobacco smoke will decrease their risk of certain cancers, they should also be taught that controlling their myopia may decrease their risk of certain eye diseases.

Glaucoma

Glaucoma is a term used to describe a group of eye diseases that cause damage to the optic nerve and can lead to partial vision loss or complete blindness. The optic nerve is a bundle of more than one million nerve fibers that connect the retina to the brain. Messages are sent through the optic nerve so your brain can interpret the things you are seeing with your eyes. A healthy optic nerve is essential to maintaining clear vision. If your optic nerve is damaged, the images being sent to your brain may become unclear.

Inside the front of the eye, there is an area called the anterior chamber. A clear fluid flows in and out of this chamber in order to nourish the eye tissue. The fluid flows out of the eye through a meshwork located where the sclera (the white part of the eye) and the iris (the colored part of the eye) meet. If for any reason, the meshwork gets blocked, and the fluid is prevented from flowing normally, the fluid can build up in the eye, causing pressure inside the eyeball. This increased pressure can push against the optic nerve, permanently damaging it.

Multiple types of glaucoma include open-angle glaucoma, normal-tension glaucoma, angle-closure glaucoma, congenital glaucoma, secondary glaucoma, pigmentary glaucoma, and pseudo-exfoliation glaucoma. The causes of these different forms of glaucoma vary, but they can all result in damage to the optic nerve. During a regular exam, your eye doctor can measure the pressure in your eye to determine if there is a need for an additional follow up or treatment.

Not all of these forms of glaucoma are directly caused by severe myopia. Still, having severe myopia greatly increases your risk. For example, pigmentary glaucoma is a hereditary condition where pigment from the eye's iris sheds off and causes the fluid drainage in the eye to slow down. Pseudoexfoliation glaucoma is caused by extra material building up on the human lens, which then sheds off. Similar to pigmentary glaucoma, pseudoexfoliation glaucoma can cause the fluid in the eye to drain slower.

Secondary glaucoma is a complication of a separate medical disease or issue. For example, diabetes or chronic inflammation can cause secondary glaucoma. Secondary glaucoma may also be a complication related to eye tumors, injuries, or surgeries. Some children are born with conditions that cause congenital glaucoma.

Angle-closure glaucoma, also known as narrow angle glaucoma or acute glaucoma, is when the angle where the meshwork is located gets blocked entirely. This leads to a sudden increase in eye pressure, which can cause pain, nausea, and blurred vision.

In low- or normal-tension glaucoma, the disease develops even though the

> My wife and I were both nearsighted until Lasik. Our children were headed down that same path. As a parent, it was important to me to help them reduce that risk of progression. As a doctor, I understand the increased medical risks of retinal detachment and glaucoma with high myopia.
>
> Dr. Michael Murphy, OD

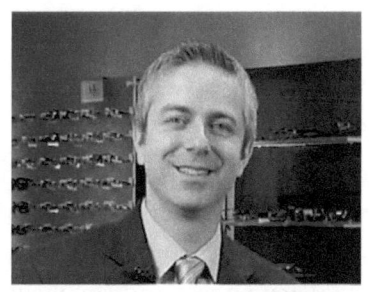

patient's eye pressure is within the normal range. The causes are not yet understood, but researchers have learned that people with a family history of the disease or with a history of systematic heart disease are at greater risk of developing it.

The most common form of glaucoma is open-angle glaucoma. With this type of glaucoma, the drainage angle is "open." This means it is not blocked or partially obstructed. In spite of that, the fluid passes through the meshwork too slowly and causes a buildup in pressure. Among other risk factors, severe and long-term myopia can contribute to open-angle glaucoma.

More than half of the people who actually have glaucoma don't know they have the disease. That is because glaucoma is typically painless even after severe damage has been done. For this reason, we recommend that everyone, not just those who have existing vision problems or those who suspect an issue, but *everyone* should get an annual eye examination. Early detection means better chances of saving your vision.

Other risk factors for developing glaucoma include:
- People who are over the age of forty
- People who have family members with glaucoma
- Those who are of African or Hispanic heritage
- Those of Asian heritage. Asians are at increased risk of angle-closure glaucoma, and those of Japanese heritage are at increased risk of low-tension glaucoma
- People who are farsighted or nearsighted
- Those who have had an eye injury
- People who have corneas that are thin in the center
- Those with diabetes, migraines, high blood pressure, poor blood circulation or other health problems affecting the whole body.

As glaucoma develops, you will slowly lose your peripheral or side vision. If it is left untreated, the side vision will continue to decrease until it feels like you are looking through a tunnel. Eventually, straight-ahead vision will start to be impacted until you are completely blind.

Glaucoma can be diagnosed through a series of eye exams, including the visual acuity test and the visual field test. These are standard tests your doctor will conduct during your annual eye exam, which test your vision at different distances and the extent of your peripheral vision. There is also the dilated eye exam, where your eye doctor puts drops in your eyes that force your pupils to dilate. This allows your doctor to see farther into the back of your eye to examine your retina and optic nerve.

Another test your eye doctor may conduct is tonometry, which measures the pressure in your eye. This can reveal the development of glaucoma or specific conditions within the eye that could lead to the development of glaucoma. There is also pachymetry, a test that measures the thickness of your cornea. This test is done using an ultrasonic wave instrument.

Advancements in technology are allowing optometrists more options when testing for glaucoma. For example, optical coherence tomography (OCT) tests provide eye doctors with a better look at the optic nerve when a glaucoma diagnosis is uncertain. Pattern electroretinography (ERG) tests may be able to detect glaucoma much earlier than previously possible. According to the National Institute of Health, "Changes in pattern ERG results can be detected approximately eight years sooner than changes in RNFL (retinal nerve fiber layer) thickness."

There is no cure for glaucoma. Once you start experiencing vision loss, that loss cannot be restored. However, there are treatments available to slow or even stop the progression of glaucoma once it is detected. These treatments include medicines, conventional surgery, laser trabeculoplasty, or a combination of these treatment options.

There are also medicines available to lower the pressure inside the eye. However, some glaucoma eye drops have been known to cause irritation, burning, or redness. It is vital that once you are prescribed a medicine for glaucoma that you continue taking it as directed by your eye doctor. As mentioned earlier, glaucoma is painless, which leads some people to believe their condition has improved. However, stopping the medicine too soon may cause your glaucoma to progress.

Conventional surgery options are available to treat glaucoma as well. During surgery, the surgeon will create a new opening for the fluid to drain from your eye. This surgery is performed on one eye at a time, with a span of four to six weeks between surgeries. Following each one, you will need to put drops in your eyes for several weeks to prevent infection. As with any surgery, there are potential complications to consider. While any loss in vision won't be restored, if successful, this surgery can stop the progression of glaucoma, preventing further vision loss. Once the new opening is created, the fluid can flow normally from the eye, which prevents further buildup of pressure.

The third treatment option is laser trabeculoplasty. This procedure uses a laser to stretch the drainage holes in the meshwork between the sclera and iris, allowing more fluid to pass through the holes. Following this surgery, you will need to be continually monitored by your eye doctor to watch for future buildup of fluid. You may also need to continue taking glaucoma medication. Although this procedure has been proven effective in many patients, the effects are not always long lasting.

An estimated $2.5 billion of the country's health care budget is spent on glaucoma annually, with patients paying an additional $1.9 billion out of pocket. Glaucoma also accounts for more than ten million doctor and emergency room visits each year. Patients with early-onset glaucoma can expect to pay an average of $623 per year, while patients with advanced glaucoma can pay as much as $2,511 per year.

According to *Glaucomatoday.com*, "Health economists estimate that more than $1.5 billion is spent on Social Security benefits, lost income tax revenue, and health care expenditures related to glaucoma." With the astronomical financial and emotional costs of this devastating eye disease, there is a clear need to take control of myopia and reduce your risk, preserving your eye health in the future.

Cataracts

Within your eye is a clear disc known as the human lens. This lens helps focus the light that enters the eye through the cornea on the retina. The retina then sends a signal to the brain to tell you what you are seeing. In order for the retina to receive a perfect image, the lens must be completely clear. A cataract happens when the lens gets cloudy, negatively affecting vision. Cataracts can form in one or both eyes. However, it is not a condition that spreads, so if it develops in both eyes, it does so independently.

The eye's lens, which is made up of water and protein, is located behind the iris and pupil. Normally, the protein is naturally arranged so that the lens stays clear. However, for a variety of reasons, the proteins in the lens can get clumpy. Groups of them can stick together, creating a cataract. Once a cataract is formed, your vision will start to become blurry. The longer it goes untreated, the more proteins will clump together, and the blurrier your vision will get. A cataract can form as a result of surgery or trauma to the eye, as well as diabetes, smoking, or simply from age.

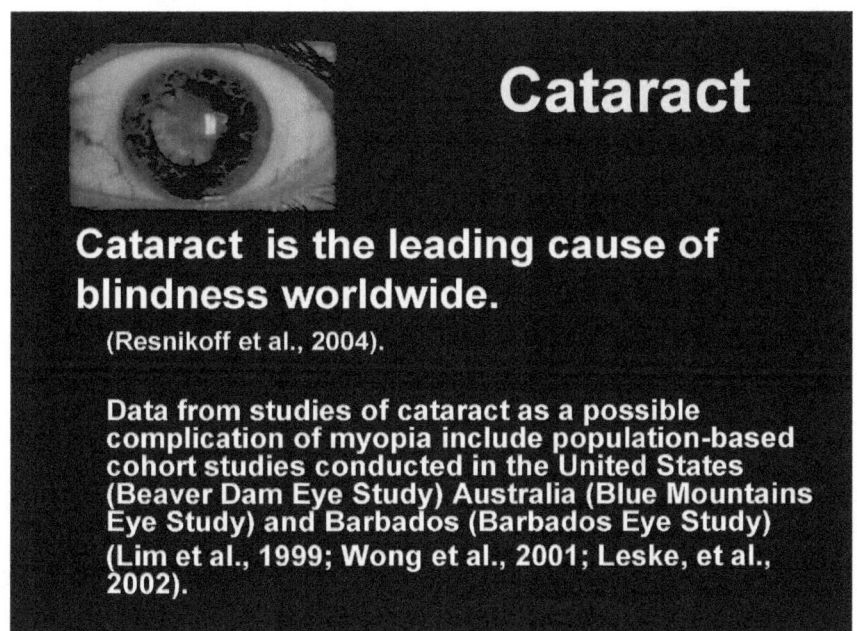

Cataract is the leading cause of blindness worldwide.
(Resnikoff et al., 2004).

Data from studies of cataract as a possible complication of myopia include population-based cohort studies conducted in the United States (Beaver Dam Eye Study) Australia (Blue Mountains Eye Study) and Barbados (Barbados Eye Study) (Lim et al., 1999; Wong et al., 2001; Leske, et al., 2002).

Cataracts are often thought of as an old person's eye disease, but this is not an accurate description. While it is true that your chances of developing cataracts increase as you age, cataracts that occur from wear and tear can start developing as young as your forties. This wear and tear includes the long-term strain caused by severe myopia. Cataract and Refractive Surgery Today's website states that, "Cataracts in severely myopic patients tend to develop at an earlier age and progress faster." The longer you have uncontrolled myopia, the more it will negatively impact your vision.

Symptoms of cataracts include blurry vision, increased glare from oncoming headlights, decreased night vision, double vision, faded colors, and frequent changes in your corrective lens prescription. When experiencing any of these symptoms, it is important to see your eye doctor as soon as possible. Your doctor will conduct a thorough eye examination in order to determine if you do, in fact, have cataracts. The eye exam will include a visual acuity test, a dilated eye exam, and tonometry. These are three of the same tests conducted to diagnose glaucoma.

"At $10.7 billion [annually], cataracts are the second costliest disorder and the most expensive medical diagnosis" (*Economic Burden of Vision Loss Report*, June 11, 2013). This expense is mostly due to the fact that surgery is the only effective treatment for cataracts. During cataract surgery, the eye surgeon removes the cloudy human lens and replaces it with a clear artificial lens. However, in the early stages of cataracts, vision can be improved by using special glasses, anti-glare sunglasses, and brighter lightening. Generally speaking, cataract surgery is not recommended until the cataracts negatively impact daily activities.

Macular Degeneration

Macular degeneration is the leading cause of vision loss in people over the age of fifty. Macular degeneration causes vision loss by damaging the macula, a small area made up of millions of light-sensing cells, located close to the center of the retina. A healthy macula provides crisp, clear central vision. It is the most sensitive part of the retina and can be affected by any damage to that area of the eye, including retinal detachments, eye injuries, and surgery.

When the macula is damaged, the center of your vision field will become blurry, distorted, and eventually, dark. You may experience a blind spot in the center of your vision field. As the degeneration progresses, the blind spot will become larger. Although a total loss of central vision may take a long time, even minor macular degeneration can interfere with normal daily activities.

With macular degeneration, you will be unable to clearly see what is immediately in front of you. This may prevent you from being able to do necessary daily activities like cooking, housework, reading, writing, and driving. It may also impede your ability to see people standing right in front of you. There are many risk factors associated with the development of macular degeneration, including age, race, smoking, and family history. Other eye diseases may also contribute to the development of macular degeneration. "For instance, in a pooled analysis of two major population-based studies, eyes which had undergone lens extraction (cataract surgery) had a 5.7-fold increased risk of developing late AMD (age-related macular degeneration)" (*www.amdbook.org*).

Similar to other eye diseases, macular degeneration is painless in the early stages. You may simply start to notice blurriness directly in front of you when trying to focus on something. Of the five tests your doctor may perform to help diagnose macular degeneration, the first two are a visual acuity test and a dilated eye exam, which will likely be conducted during your annual eye exam. Your doctor may also have you look at an Amsler grid to ensure you can see all the lines on the grid. Damage to the macula can cause some of the lines to disappear or look wavy.

The next test, a fluorescein angiogram, must be performed by an ophthalmologist as it involves the eye being injected with a fluorescent dye. The doctor will then take a picture as the dye works its way through the eye's blood vessels. This will show any possible blood vessel leakages in the eye. The fifth test is an optical coherence tomography (OCT) and utilizes light waves to get high-resolution images of the eye tissue.

While examining your eyes, your eye doctor will also look for something called drusen. These are yellow deposits of lipids that develop below the retina. Most people develop small drusen as they age. However, medium or large deposits of these lipids may be a sign of macular degeneration. The identification of drusen allows your eye doctor to determine at which stage of macular degeneration you are in. Early macular degeneration is diagnosed when medium-sized drusen are found. During early macular degeneration, patients typically haven't experienced any vision loss yet.

With intermediate macular degeneration, you may start to experience blurriness and some vision loss. During this stage, your eye doctor will likely find large drusen and/or pigment changes in the retina. However, these changes won't be visible to the patient. These two symptoms can only be found through a comprehensive eye exam, which is another reason to make sure you schedule regular exams. Catching the disease before or during the intermediate stage when full vision may still be present is essential.

The third stage is late macular degeneration, and there are two forms. The first, geographic atrophy, is when the light-sensitive cells in the macula break down, causing vision loss. The second, neovascular macular degeneration, or wet macular degeneration, is when abnormal blood vessels grow under the retina and

> One of the great things about Ortho K is that it slows down the worsening of my vision over time. With glasses, I would have to keep getting new prescriptions every six months. For the Ortho K retainers, I only have to change it a little bit each year. My eyes aren't getting as bad so I can keep that 20/20 vision.
>
> **~ Kevin Heath**
> **Patient of Dr. Page**

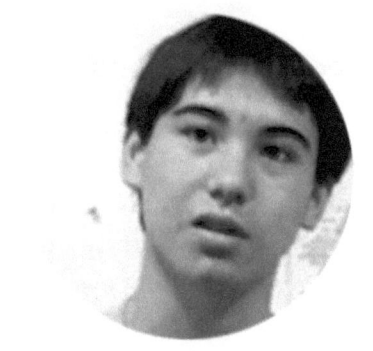

leak blood into the macula, causing vision loss. Until there is vision loss, most people experience no symptoms that indicate they are developing macular degeneration.

As with glaucoma, once you experience vision loss, that vision cannot be restored. A few medications are believed to slow the progression of vision loss due to macular degeneration. Depending on the medication, it will need to be given anywhere from once a month to once every two months. The National Eye Institute also recommends specific vitamins and minerals for the treatment and prevention of macular degeneration. Vitamin C, Vitamin E, beta-carotene, zinc, and copper have all been shown to slow the progression of vision loss in patients.

In addition to medications or supplements, patients may be eligible for a surgical procedure. Laser photocoagulation cauterizes leaking blood vessels, thus stopping the leakage. This laser treatment is effective in 10 percent to 20 percent of patients. The downside to this procedure, even when it is effective, is that it will create scar tissue on the eye that will appear as blind spots in the patient's vision.

There are also drug treatments available that have been shown to provide good results. Lucentis and Avastin are both drugs that can be injected into the eye for the treatment of macular degeneration. Although these drugs are still fairly new and have shown great promise, they can be costly. In 2012, the *New York Times* reported that, "One of the most heavily reimbursed procedures—costing a total of $1 billion for 143,000 patients—is for a single treatment for an eye disorder common in the elderly"—age-related macular degeneration. Some professionals have gone as far as to call these miracle drugs because they are the first drugs available that have the potential to reverse some of the vision loss caused by macular degeneration.

Other Complications

In addition to these eye diseases, severe myopia also causes eyestrain. Eyestrain can lead to chronic fatigue and headaches. It can also cause eye irritation and dryness. These complications, along with the poor vision of myopia, can significantly impact your quality of life and your ability to work. Dealing with ongoing eye irritation and dryness can make it uncomfortable to wear contact lenses. It can also negatively impact your tear production, which can lead to dry eye disease. Although dry eye disease can be treated with special eye drops, it can lead to an increased risk of eye infections and scarring on the eye's surface.

Glaucoma, cataracts, and macular degeneration aren't the only health complications associated with severe myopia. You are also at a significantly increased risk of retinal detachment. The more severe your myopia, the greater your risk of retinal tearing, holes, and eventually, detachment. Just having a prescription of -4.0D increases your risk of retinal detachment by as much as one thousand times. These risks will be discussed in greater detail in the next chapter.

Controlling your child's myopia will decrease their risk of developing these eye diseases and help to preserve their vision as they age. Obviously, myopia is not the only risk factor associated with eye diseases. Other common risk factors include age, gender, ethnicity, certain medications, inadequate exposure to natural sunlight, and the use of electronic devices. While some of these factors are more difficult, if not impossible to control, myopia is one that can be.

Although the research determining the extent of the risk myopia presents is still ongoing, all of the research conducted to date proves a link between severe myopia and the development of eye diseases. As the current generation of children ages, there will be a dramatic spike in glaucoma, cataracts, macular degeneration, and retinal detachment if more is not done to control myopia.

CHAPTER THREE

How Myopia Can Lead to Retinal Detachment

Many of the eye diseases discussed in the previous chapter negatively impact the cornea or the optic nerve. However, the retina, a light-sensitive thin layer of tissue that lines the inside of the eye, is just as vital to vision. Light penetrates through the lens, which projects images of the world onto the retina. The retina then sends messages via chemical and electrical signals down the optic nerve, so the brain can identify what is being seen.

In certain situations the retina can become detached from the inside of the eye, causing loss of vision. This happens when the retina is lifted or pulled away from the inside wall. Even if only a small portion of the retina pulls away, it is still considered a detachment. The retina can also be stretched as the eye elongates to a point where it tears and holes forms, which is how the progression of myopia can cause retinal detachment.

There are four types of retinal detachment. The first type is called Rhegmatogenous. This is the most common form of retinal detachment and happens when a tear or break forms in the retina, allowing fluid to get under the retinal layer. The fluid then lifts the retina, forcing it to detach from the inside wall of the eye. Another type of retinal detachment is called Tractional. This occurs when scar tissue on the surface of the retina contracts, causing the retina to separate. The third type is called Exudative. This type of retinal detachment is typically caused by a retinal disease or sudden eye injury. Although it doesn't involve an actual tear or hole, fluid is still able to get under the retina. Proliferative vitreoretinopathy, the last form of retinal detachment, is a complication that can occur after retinal detachment surgery. As the retina heals from surgery, cells form on the surface, causing the retina to detach again.

How Myopia Can Lead to Retinal Detachment

There are a number of things that can cause retinal detachments and a number of factors that can increase the risk. Some of these factors include having already had a retinal detachment in that eye, a family history of retinal detachment, cataract surgery, an eye injury, or an eye disease such as degenerative myopia.

Degenerative myopia is nearsightedness that continues to progress rapidly. According to an article published by the Contact Lens Spectrum, the risk associated with degenerative myopia "is not linear but is related to the level of refractive error, starting at 0.3% for very low myopia (–1.00D) and rising to 3.0% for moderate myopia (–3.00D to –5.00D), 28.6% for high myopia (–7.00D to –9.00D), and 52.4% for very high myopia (> –9.00D). In fact, for every –0.25D myopia increase, this risk becomes 17% higher." This is due to the elongation of the eyeball. As the eye stretches from myopia, more stress is applied to the retina, which causes it to weaken. That constant stress and weakening over time causes the retina to detach or begin to tear.

If you suspect you might have a detached retina, it is extremely important to get to an eye doctor or emergency room immediately. There is a very small window of time in which an eye doctor can reattach your retina and save your vision. The symptoms of retinal detachment include seeing an increase in the specks, threads, or what look like little cobwebs that *float* through your vision, and sudden light flashes. Another common symptom is a darkening of your peripheral vision—what many describe as a curtain falling or closing over your field of vision.

There are two common treatments for retinal tears. The first is laser surgery. During the procedure, the

> I have been wearing the overnight contact lens since I was 10 years old. Ortho-K is just perfect for me. I am a dancer and swimmer, and wearing glasses can be very inconvenient and awkward. With Ortho-k, I am able to see everything clearly without glasses. The thought of never having to wear glasses or contacts is very liberating! Thank you very much Dr. Page. I am very grateful to you and your amazing team.
>
> ~ Monet

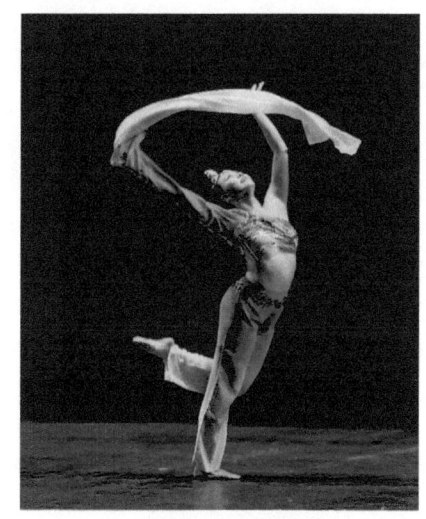

doctor will use a laser to burn the area around the tear. This creates scar tissue that *welds* the retina to the under tissue of the inside of the eyeball. The second option is called cryopexy, which involves freezing the retinal tear. The doctor will position a probe over the tear and freeze the area around the hole. Similar to laser surgery, this process will create scar tissue holding the retina to the underlying layers of the eyeball.

For a full retinal detachment, where the retina is pulling away or lifting from the inside wall of the eye, there are two options for treatment. The first, called a vitrectomy, involves injecting air or gas into the eye. The doctor first removes the vitreous, the gel-like fluid that fills the interior of the eyeball, and replaces it with air. The bubble of air then presses against the retina and pushes it back into place. As the eye heals, it creates more vitreous fluid that slowly replaces the air.

The second treatment option uses a scleral buckle, which is a thin silicone band. The buckle is sewn to the sclera, the white part of the eyeball, so it will gently indent the wall of the eye, relieving the pressure being put in the retina. In both treatments, laser surgery or cryopexy are used to secure the retina back into place. Currently, research is being conducted on the use of silicone oil in combination with long-acting intraocular gas for the treatment of proliferative vitreoretinopathy-type retinal detachments.

According to the National Eye Institute's website, "With modern therapy, over 90 percent of those with a retinal detachment can be successfully treated, although sometimes a second treatment is needed. However, the visual outcome is not always predictable… Even under the best of circumstances, and even after multiple attempts at repair, treatment sometimes fails and vision may eventually be lost."

As myopia progresses, the retina will continue to stretch, causing even greater elongation. It is this elongation of the retina that affects your vision. The longer the eye gets, the more stress is put on various areas of the eyeball. As mentioned in the previous chapter, myopia not only puts stress on the optic nerve, which can contribute to glaucoma, but it can also put stress on the retina, potentially causing it to stretch, tear, and eventually detach.

Currently, myopia-related retinal detachment is fairly uncommon. However, this is likely due to the fact that the number of older people who had progressive myopia is relatively low. With the increase in the prevalence of myopia hitting younger and younger generations, the more the prevalence of retinal detachments will increase.

How Myopia Can Lead to Retinal Detachment

In countries like China, where the prevalence of myopia is as high as 90 percent in some areas, citizens will soon be faced with a serious epidemic. "One of their concerns is myopic retinopathy in high myopia (defined as over -6.0D of myopia)" (*Erasmusmc.nl*). While retinal detachment can be successfully treated if caught early enough, undetected it can quickly lead to vision loss. Many people don't know what to look for with a retinal detachment, and since there is no pain involved, they often don't see a doctor until it is too late.

As mentioned previously, symptoms that may indicate a retinal detachment are present, but many people are either unaware of what the symptoms are or choose to ignore them. Some may assume symptoms like the sudden flashes of light aren't real, mistaking them for car headlights or lightning. For example, I once had a patient who had her retina detach while she was out to dinner with her husband and a couple of close friends. During dinner, she started complaining about there being flies everywhere. She got so upset about the flies floating around her food that she got up and went to the bathroom. When she did, she realized the flies she kept seeing moved with her. She had her husband take her to the emergency room, and they discovered that her retina had detached.

This patient was seeing what many people call floaters—small spots that move in and out of your vision field. For some people, they may have noticed floaters before, so the sudden appearance of more floaters or the larger size of the floaters is not alarming to them. However, any changes in your vision field, whether they be floaters, light flashes, or a darkening in your peripheral vision, should be checked out immediately by an eye doctor as they could be a symptom of retinal detachment. Even when the retina is successfully reattached, the scarring from the initial injury or from the subsequent surgery can cause permanent vision loss. The National Eye Institute recommends that "Visual results are best if the retinal detachment is repaired before the macula (the center region of the retina responsible for fine, detailed vision) detaches." So again, early detection is key.

Recovering from retinal detachment surgery can involve weeks of bed rest. Although there are newer and better options for treatment, as with any surgery there are risks involved. We will discuss the risks and side effects of corrective surgery in the following chapter.

As with the risks inherent with the eye diseases described in the previous chapter, once there is vision loss, that vision cannot be recovered. Currently, there is no surgery or medicine that can restore vision lost due to a retinal detachment. The hope with surgery is simply to save what vision is still there.

Since the retina weakens due to the stress placed on it from the elongation of the eyeball, controlling your myopia may reduce your risks of developing a detached retina. If the eyeball stops elongating, no further stress is being put on the retina and the risk of it stretching and tearing decreases significantly.

With the rise in the prevalence of myopia, it is expected that the prevalence of retinal detachment will also rise. As such, it is highly likely that the number of individuals living with full or partial blindness will also increase dramatically as the younger generations age. This will in turn lead to an increase in healthcare costs nationwide, unless we do something to stop the prevalence of myopia now.

CHAPTER FOUR

Corrective Eye Surgery

There are currently three options for treating myopia. The first and most common solution is to wear daily corrective lenses in the form of either glasses or contacts. The second is myopia control, which is the theme of this book and what we will delve into in later chapters. The third is corrective eye surgery. There are two common types of laser eye surgery intended to correct myopia—LASIK and PRK. In addition, there is a variation of PRK known as LASEK, which is less common but still available.

A surgical procedure called ICL is also available, but it is usually only used as an option for patients who are not good candidates for the other types of laser eye surgery. Finally, there is a new procedure called Kamra Inlay, which is unlike all of the other surgical options currently available. Each of these eye surgery options comes with its own host of advantages and disadvantages. Understanding the risks of each can help you make an informed and clear decision regarding which solution is right for you.

LASIK surgery has become very popular and more accessible over recent years. It is the most recent version of laser surgery, a technique developed after PRK. Due to the shorter recovery time, many patients with myopia prefer LASIK. They see it as an immediate and lasting solution to their nearsightedness. However, there are many things about LASIK surgery that are important to understand before considering it.

LASIK

When looking at options to permanently "fix" their blurred vision caused by myopia, many people look at LASIK eye surgery. The word *LASIK* is an acronym which stands for laser-assisted in-situ keratomileusis. LASIK is a type of refractive surgery, a procedure that uses lasers to change the shape of the cornea. The purpose of refractive surgery is to reshape the cornea, forcing the light rays that enter the eye to bend and focus on the retina to create clearer, crisper vision. LASIK is the most commonly practiced refractive surgery. It can be used to treat myopia, hyperopia, and astigmatism.

During the surgery, the eye surgeon will cut a thin flap from the cornea. The flap is folded back so the surgeon can get to the underlying tissue, also called the stromal layer. The surgeon then uses an excimer laser to burn away some of the tissue. The amount of corneal tissue removed is microscopic, just enough to reshape the cornea so light can be focused on the retina.

In myopic patients, the surgeon will flatten the cornea in order to focus the light on the retina correctly, improving the clarity of the patient's vision. For hyperopic patients (people with farsightedness), the shape of cornea needs to be steeper. When dealing with astigmatisms, the surgeon will use the laser to smooth out the irregular shape of the cornea. After the cornea is reshaped, the flap is put back into place, covering the area where the tissue was burned away. The cornea will heal on its own, without needing any stitches or bandages, but patients are provided with topical anesthetic drops for pain.

Before performing the surgery, your eye surgeon will need to determine whether or not you are a good candidate for LASIK. This includes performing an eye exam to analyze the shape and thickness of the cornea, and determine refractive errors and pupil size. The doctor will also examine the moistness of your eyes since dryness is one of the risks associated with the surgery.

The surgeon will then map the shape of your eye using an instrument called a corneal topographer. This allows him or her to examine the surface shape and curvature of the cornea. The doctor will also conduct a wave-front analysis, which uses light waves to examine any aberrations that are impacting your vision. Finally, the surgeon will examine your general health history and look at any medications you are currently taking.

Before the surgery begins, you can expect to have numbing drops put in your eyes to eliminate any pain or discomfort during the procedure. An instrument called the lid speculum is used to hold your eye open. The surgeon will use a special type of ink to mark the cornea prior to cutting the flap. After the flap is cut and folded back, the surgeon will adjust the laser as needed and ask you to look at a specific target. While you maintain your focus on that target, the surgeon will send laser pulses at your cornea, reshaping it.

The surgery usually lasts about five minutes per eye. Many patients say they feel pressure on their eye during surgery, but not any pain due to the numbing drops. When the procedure is complete, the surgeon will have you recover for an hour or two in the office before performing a post-operative eye exam.

You may experience blurry or hazy vision immediately following the procedure, as well as a burning or itching sensation. While these are normal, they should go away after the first day. If not, you will need to see your eye doctor immediately. In most cases, you can return to work and your normal activities the next day, waiting about a week before doing anything too strenuous.

If successful, LASIK surgery can provide 20/20 vision. However, there are risks and potential complications to consider. LASIK surgery isn't always successful. In some cases, your vision may be improved but not enough to eliminate the need for corrective lenses. The surgeon may also need to go back and do the surgery again after a couple of months. This is often referred to as a *touch-up* or enhancement procedure. Even with the touch-up surgery, you may still have to wear reading glasses after having the procedure.

As with any surgery, there are several risks and potential complications with LASIK. Therefore, "you are probably not a good candidate for refractive surgery if you are not a risk taker" (www.fda.gov). One of the risks is under-correction, which is when the surgeon does not remove enough tissue from the cornea. This results in not having the crisp, clear vision you hoped you would get from the surgery. Under-corrections are typically when touch-up procedures are needed and is most common with myopic patients.

Another potential risk is overcorrection, wherein the surgeon removes too much tissue from the cornea. Due to the permanent nature of the surgery, over-corrections cannot be completely fixed. Once the tissue is removed, it cannot be put back.

While LASIK eye surgery can be used to eliminate astigmatism, if the tissue from the eye is not removed evenly (symmetrically), it can create astigmatism. Depending on how much tissue is removed, it may or may not be possible to correct the creation of astigmatism. Additional surgery may be needed or the patient may need to wear corrective lenses. Although the percentage of cases is low, it is not uncommon for patients of LASIK to have to go back to wearing glasses or contacts.

Another risk to laser eye surgery is that your vision quality may return to what it was prior to the procedure. In a study of postoperative patients, "at two months and two years, 83 percent of eyes were within +/- 1.00D, which decreased to 42 percent at seven to eight years" (www.ncbi.nlm.nih.gov). While LASIK surgery may "correct" your current myopia, it does not stop the progression of it. This means that your eyes can still develop myopia after the surgery. The development of myopia can be impacted by abnormal healing, pregnancy, or other hormonal imbalances, as well as the same conditions that caused the myopia initially, such as the use of electronic devices and too much close work. In such cases, you may have to go back to wearing glasses or contacts. Redoing the procedure may not be an option, depending on how much tissue was removed during the initial surgery.

Other risks and complications you may experience include infection, dryness, irritation, corneal scarring resulting in permanent damage to the shape of the cornea (which makes wearing contact lenses impossible), a decrease in contrast sensitivity (even if 20/20 vision is achieved, objects may still blend together or look fuzzy), glares or haloes resulting in problems with driving at night, double vision, light sensitivity, and reduced or permanent vision loss.

Glares or haloes occur when viewing bright lights, particularly at night. Lights, such as those from oncoming cars, may cause you to see haloes around the light source or a great deal of glare, impairing your field of vision. Additionally, your quality of vision at dusk or in other dim light conditions may be worse than it was before you had the surgery. These complications can make driving in the evenings or at night difficult and dangerous.

LASIK surgery can also cause irritation and dry eyes. For approximately six months following the procedure, you may experience a decrease in tear production. This can make your eyes feel dry and itchy. It can also negatively impact your quality of vision. Depending on the severity of your dryness, you may be prescribed special eye drops or need to have a second surgery to keep your tears on the surface of your eyes as opposed to them draining away.

In addition to other complications such as infections, inflammation, and excessive tear production, you may also experience ongoing problems if the corneal flap created during surgery heals improperly, which can impair your vision. As a result of LASIK, some patients experience partial or full loss of vision. Although rare, in those cases, the patients' vision is worse following the procedure. Due to the permanent nature of the surgery, once the vision is lost, it cannot be restored.

According to a 2014 report issued by the FDA, 45 percent of patients experienced haloes, glare, starbursts, and ghosting following their LASIK eye surgery. Yet, these individuals did not experience such symptoms prior to having the surgery. Thirty percent of the patients studied experienced dry eye following their LASIK surgery, but had no symptoms of dry eye prior to surgery. Another study published in the "Journal of Cataract and Refractive Surgery," provided the following statistics. Of the patients included in the study, 50 percent experienced ongoing irritation, 43 percent experienced glare, 41 percent experienced haloes, and 35.2 percent reported having trouble seeing in dim light.

While no surgery is without complications, the risks associated with LASIK surgery are fairly common. LASIK surgery is permanent, so if the surgery is unsuccessful or creates unintended outcomes, it cannot be reversed. In some cases, additional surgeries can help correct the complications, but those procedures come with additional risks as well. While vision loss is referred to by many in the industry as a rare complication, it is still a risk and one that should not be taken lightly.

In addition to the potential complications of LASIK eye surgery, it is important to understand that this surgery does not control or prevent the progression of myopia. Since LASIK surgery does not correct the elongation of the eyeball, your vision can still worsen after the surgery, putting you at an even greater risk of eye disease later in life.

> As an active 7th grader, I like to play tennis. When I wore glasse, they didn't really work for me because they'd slip off my face when I was running around the court. Contacts would irritate my eyes during the day, and I'd have to take them out to clean them. It was just really a big hastle. Now, I wear the these things called Ortho K braces. Dr. Page helped me find the right pair to wear every night and I take them out in the morning. I can see perfectly, and it's really nice.
>
> ~ Anderson
> Patient of Dr Page

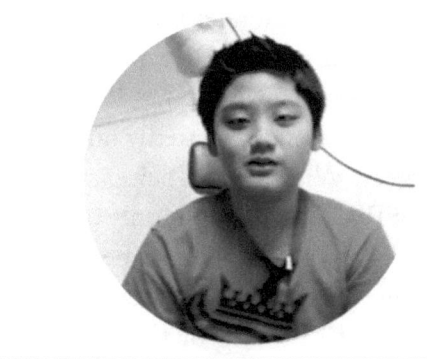

As with any elective surgery, not everyone is a good candidate for LASIK surgery. According to the U.S. National Library of Medicine's website, "LASIK may not be recommended for patients with diabetes, rheumatoid arthritis, lupus, glaucoma, herpes infections of the eye, or cataracts." If your myopia is severe, the elongation of the cornea may be too much to safely remove any tissue.

LASIK surgery also isn't recommended for people with mild myopia, such as children, due to the fact that myopia continues to progress in most patients, and the procedure can only be performed if the patient's condition is stable. With mild myopic patients, the potential risks of LASIK eye surgery often outweigh the benefits.

PRK

The second option in laser eye surgery is PRK, which stands for photorefractive keratectomy. Like LASIK, PRK can be used to correct myopia, hyperopia, and astigmatism. Although it is the predecessor to LASIK eye surgery, it is still widely used. PRK was the first version of laser eye surgery designed to correct vision. Unlike LASIK, instead of creating a flap before reshaping the cornea, with PRK surgery, the entire outer layer of the cornea, called the epithelium, is removed. This exposes the stromal layer, which is the layer of the cornea that is reshaped with the excimer laser.

Both types of laser eye surgery essentially do the same thing by reshaping the same area of the cornea to bend light toward the retina. The main difference is how much of the epithelial tissue is cut or removed. Since the entire epithelium is removed during PRK, the recovery time is longer than with LASIK because the epithelial cells need time to regenerate.

In addition to a longer recovery time, there is a slight increase in the risk of post-operative infection. PRK patients also experience slightly more discomfort, and their vision typically takes longer to stabilize. The final results regarding the quality of vision can actually take several weeks to become evident following PRK surgery. With all that being said, it seems that LASIK would be the clear choice, yet PRK is still commonly used. Despite these drawbacks, there are clear benefits to PRK surgery for some patients.

As your myopia progresses the eyeball elongates, which results in the stretching and thinning of the retina. In order to have laser eye surgery, the cornea needs to be thick enough that some of the tissue can be removed during the reshaping process. Not creating a flap, as is done in LASIK, leaves more of the stromal tissue intact to reshape. For patients with severe myopia, the cornea may not be thick enough to make them good candidates for LASIK surgery, leaving them with the option of PRK surgery.

Additional benefits of PRK include the elimination of complications associated with the corneal flap not healing correctly. This surgery also reduces the risk of overcorrection (removing too much of the cornea with the laser). PRK is also an option for patients who have already had LASIK surgery and do not have enough corneal tissue for a follow-up surgery.

LASEK

LASEK is a combination of PRK and LASIK techniques. It is not as commonly used as the other two, but it is still an option to consider when looking into corrective surgery. Similar to PRK surgery, LASEK is more ideal for patients who are not good candidates for LASIK due to the thickness of their cornea.

The basic difference between this surgery and the other two is how the eye is prepped for the procedure. As mentioned earlier, LASIK involves creating a flap in the epithelium, while PRK involves removing the entire layer. During LASEK surgery, the epithelial tissue is separated and pushed to the side, exposing the stromal layer. After the cornea is reshaped, the thin layer of epithelium is pulled back over the eye. This allows it to heal quickly, but also allows the eye surgeon to remove a thinner slice of tissue than in LASIK, so it is a viable option for more patients.

When comparing LASEK to the other two methods, LASEK's advantage over LASIK is that it eliminates complications related to the flap healing incorrectly. As with PRK, LASEK decreases the risk of overcorrection (removing too much of the cornea). There is also a lower risk of developing dry eye following LASEK surgery. Unlike PRK, LASEK surgery preserves the epithelium.

Although the theoretical advantage of this technique was intended to be faster recovery times, many eye surgeons have found no reduction in how long it takes for the eye to heal. Some even argue that recovery takes longer with LASEK than PRK. Due to the unclear benefit of LASEK over PRK, PRK is still the preferred method.

ICL

The fourth surgery option, which uses a laser but is not considered laser surgery, is an implantable contact lens or ICL. This surgery is considered an outpatient procedure and generally takes less than fifteen minutes. The lens inserted in the eye is called the Visian ICL, and is made of a collagen copolymer product called collamer.

Once inserted, the lens cannot be felt or seen by the patient. Collagen is already a naturally occurring substance in the eye, so the collamer mimics the eye's natural feel. The Visian ICL also has a built-in ultraviolet filter to protect the eye when exposed to sunlight. The lens is implanted just behind the iris, in front of the eye's natural lens.

Candidates for ICL have to be between the ages of twenty-one and forty-five. They have to be nearsighted (of -3.0D to -20.0D) with little to no astigmatism. The patient's eye needs to have adequate anterior chamber depth (the space between the iris and the endothelium or the cornea's inner surface) and eye tissue cell density in order to accommodate the ICL. This is something your ophthalmologist will determine during your eye examination. Your vision needs to have been stable for at least a year prior to the surgery. Generally, patients considered for ICL are not good candidates for laser eye surgery. Based on recovery time, LASIK surgery is recommended over ICL. However, because no part of the eye is being removed, ICL can work for patients who are ineligible for LASIK due to severe nearsightedness, thin corneas, or severe dry eye.

In addition to providing an option for those patients not eligible for LASIK surgery, ICL has several other benefits. It typically does not cause dry eye syndrome, which is a concern with laser eye surgeries. ICL provides sharp vision with increased night vision. The lens provides UV protection, the procedure is relatively short, and you can see the benefits within a couple of days. Another benefit is that the lens can be removed if need be through an additional surgery. While no one wants to go through multiple surgeries if they don't have to, in most cases the lenses can be removed without damaging your eyes if you decide you no longer want them for any reason. Unlike laser surgery, the changes are not permanent.

As with laser eye surgery, the surgeon will use a topical anesthetic to numb the eye before beginning ICL surgery. The surgeon will then create a couple of small openings at the bottom of your cornea. A gel solution is used to protect your eye while the lens is being positioned. Another small opening is created and the Visian ICL is inserted just beneath your eye's natural lens. You may feel pressure during the procedure. The lens is rectangular but the four corners are positioned behind your iris, so the lens is not visible to anyone.

The incisions made to insert and place the lens are so small that stitches are generally not needed. Your doctor will provide you with eye drops to prevent an infection while you recover. You may also get an eye patch to wear the first couple of nights to ensure you don't rub or scratch your eye. Just like with any other surgical procedure, there is a risk of infection, but it is minimal so long as you use the eye drops as prescribed. Similar to laser eye surgery, there are also the risks of over- or under-correction, haloes, and night glare with ICL. These are risks you will need to take into consideration with any corrective eye surgery.

In a three-year clinical trial, 99 percent of the patients who underwent ICL surgery were either satisfied or very satisfied with the results. Following the surgeries, the patients' vision were stable over the course of the three-year study. Also, the occurrence of double vision, haloes, glare, and night-driving problems were consistent from before to after the surgery, which means the surgery did not create any of these problems or make them worse. However, "cataract has been suggested to be an important long-term complication of ICL implantation" (archopht.jamanetwork.com).

While research has shown that ICL patients demonstrated stable vision for three years following the procedure, there is no evidence that it stops the progression of myopia over time. This means that your vision could worsen, resulting in the need for another ICL surgery to implant stronger lenses or the need to wear corrective lenses along with the implanted lenses. However, ICL is a viable option for patients who are not good candidates for other methods of myopia control due to the condition of their eyes.

Although not currently available in the United States, there have been advancements in the technology of these lenses in recent years that will make this procedure a viable option for patients with astigmatism up to 4.0 diopters.

KAMRA Inlay

KAMRA inlay is a relatively new procedure that partially restores a natural range of vision and reduces the patient's reliance on corrective lenses. Used mainly for presbyopic patients (people who have lost their near vision naturally as they aged), the thin ring-like implant is placed in only one eye. Similar to bifocals, that eye then becomes the *reading* eye, while the other retains its distance vision. The eyes work together to allow you to see clear at all ranges. Smaller and thinner than a regular daily contact, the inlay is implanted in front of the iris in the inner layers of the cornea. The pinhole opening in the center of the ring focuses the light entering the eye, allowing for clearer near vision.

The procedure for KAMRA inlay takes approximately twenty minutes. As with laser eye surgery, you are awake for the entire procedure, but the doctor will put numbing drops in your eye, so you won't feel anything. You will be asked to focus on a bright light while the surgeon uses a laser to make a small pocket in the inner layers of the cornea. The KAMRA inlay is then inserted into the pocket and centered over your pupil.

During the first two days following the procedure, you may experience light sensitivity, watery eyes, and eye irritation. However, most people are able to return to normal activity after the first two days. Better vision should be noticeable within the first week following the procedure. The degree of improvement varies, but some patients report a dramatic difference while others may experience fluctuations in their vision over the first six months following the surgery.

The potential side effects of the KAMRA inlay include dry eye, glare, haloes, and poor night vision. These are treatable and in most cases, do not last. There is also a chance you will still need to wear reading glasses for small print following the procedure. KAMRA inlay is still a relatively new procedure, so the long-term results and complications of the implant are not yet fully understood.

As discussed earlier in this chapter, your vision can continue to worsen as you age, even after undergoing any of these types of eye surgery. While these corrective surgery options may fix your myopia now, none of them are able to stop the progression of it. There are also no guarantees eye surgery will work for you, that it won't cause complications or make your vision worse, possibly even causing permanent vision loss. Regardless of the outcome, in most cases your eye doctor cannot reverse what has been done, especially with laser eye surgery. While ICL is reversible, and comes with fewer complications than laser eye surgery, it is only reversible through an additional surgery. The KAMRA Inlay website states that "During the clinical study, after removal of the inlay, vision generally returned to the level the patient had prior to the implantation with the KAMRA inlay. However, this does not guarantee that your vision will return to exactly what it was before surgery or that your eye will not have permanent damage."

With all the potential risks, complications, and side effects of corrective surgery, it is a wonder anyone would voluntarily undergo such a procedure, especially when there is a better and safer alternative available. Just like glasses or contact lenses, corrective surgery may give you clear vision now, but none of these options stop the progression of myopia. In some cases, they can actually make myopia worse, accelerating the development of eye diseases and retinal detachment. In the next chapter, we will discuss some of the other risks that affect myopia, causing the condition to progress further if ignored.

CHAPTER FIVE

Major Risk Factors for Developing Myopia

Many myopic patients consider their vision problems to be a fact of life, something that happens as they age. They don't recognize that it is not only heredity or age that plays a factor, but other elements as well. Some of their lifestyle choices, their job, or even where they live can all contribute to the development of myopia.

In the previous chapters, we discussed the risks that can occur as a result of myopia, from eye diseases and macular degeneration to retinal detachment. While understanding the risks of myopia is important, it is equally important to understand how myopia can develop to begin with. Only by educating parents about these risk factors can we hope to stop the rise in prevalence of myopia in younger generations.

Myopia is when light entering the eye is focused in front of the retina instead of directly on it, making distant objects appear out of focus. This occurs through axial elongation (a lengthening from front to back) of the eyeball, having a greater anterior chamber depth (a cornea that is too steeply curved), or a combination of both. So then, how does the cornea become too steeply curved or the eyeball too long?

Myopiacontrol.org states "that a complex mix of genetic and environment factors are involved." The genetic side includes heredity, ethnicity, gender, and age, all of which can affect the curvature of your cornea, while the environmental side is more extensive. Researchers recognize that geography, sunlight exposure, socioeconomic status, education level, and prolonged near work all play a role in the development of myopia.

Sunlight Exposure

Geography or where you live can cause you to develop myopia for several reasons, one of which pertains to the level at which your eyes are exposed to natural sunlight. While ultraviolet radiation (light waves "beyond" the violet end of the visible light spectrum) from sunlight is known to damage the eyes, there are visual benefits to sunlight exposure.

A 2007 study published in the *Investigative Ophthalmology and Visual Science Journal* asserted that it isn't so much what children are doing that is increasing the prevalence of myopia, but rather the amount of time they are spending indoors as opposed to outdoors. The researchers of this study followed 524 emmetropic students (meaning their vision was within normal refractive conditions) from third grade through to their eighth grade year. During that time, the researchers had the students' parents record the number of hours their children spent doing various activities, as well as their eye prescription as determined during a yearly exam.

A prescription of -0.75D or more is considered myopic. Of the 524 students, 26 percent became myopic by their eighth grade year. Based on the survey results, the most significant difference between the students who became myopic and those who did not was the amount of time they spent outside or playing outdoor sports. According to this study, the students who did not become myopic spent an average of 11.65 hours outside each week, while the students who did become nearsighted spent an average of only 7.98 hours outside each week.

Exposure to natural sunlight has been found to trigger a release of retinal dopamine, which is a neurotransmitter that helps photoreceptor cells respond to

> My daughter, who is 12 years old, is a patient of Dr. Page and Arizona's Vision. She's an active young girl, who enjoys singing, dancing, acting and anything fun. Her near-sightedness and wearing glasses has caused much discomfort for her. About 2 years ago, we decided to try Ortho-K. We have been extremely happy with her results. It has been life-changing, and she can now do anything she wants without the restriction of the glasses. She is able to focus her attention on the things that she loves to do the most.
>
> ~ Kayla King

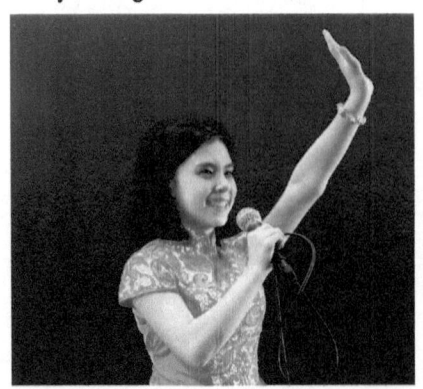

light stimulus. Studies have shown that when those dopamine levels drop, the eye enters a cycle of growth. This is when the axial of the eye lengthens, causing myopia. There has been a significant number of studies showing the relationship between dopamine levels and eye development. However, most of the research conducted has focused on the developing eyes of babies and children, so it is still unclear as to how dopamine levels impact adult eyes.

Where you live not only affects the development of myopia due to the level of sunlight exposure, but also by reducing the range of distance vision. For example, if you reside in a large city, being constantly surrounded by towering buildings reduces your level of sunlight exposure. The tightly packed buildings can also obstruct your view and decrease the distance at which your eyes can focus.

Prolonged Near Work

Probably the most contributing environmental factor is prolonged near work. This includes many lifestyle choices from what jobs we do or hobbies we enjoy. Near work can be categorized as everything from reading and writing, to sewing, knitting, drawing, and tying fishing lures—anything that involves detailed focus at close range. These activities require the eyes to focus on a close object for extended periods of time, causing the eyes to stretch and elongate.

One of the biggest culprits of prolonged near work is screen time. Research has proven a direct correlation between the recent increase in myopia prevalence and the introduction of computers and other electronic devices into our societies. Vision Council of America statistics state that more than 10 million Americans suffer from vision problems related to extended computer use.

Constantly focusing on a screen that is often too close to your face causes the eyeball to stretch as it tries to accommodate. Yet generations of young people have been staring at screens their entire lives. More and more adults have jobs that involve sitting at a computer for long periods of time. When they are not working or doing school work on a computer, both children and adults are staring at their smart phones, tablets, eReaders, or televisions. These activities not only keep their eyes focused on objects that are at close range, but they also keep them inside, which means they are relying less and less on their distance vision and not exposing their eyes to natural sunlight.

The Blue Light Hazard

The negative effects of screen time are not limited to just the prolonged amount of time spent on them. The light these screens give off also contributes to myopia and other eye problems. Light-emitting diodes, or LEDs, emit light from the blue part of the visible light spectrum. Modern electronic devices use LEDs as they don't give off as much heat as light waves from the red end of the visible light spectrum and thus, use less energy, making their battery life longer. However, blue light is the next door neighbor to ultraviolet radiation.

Because of blue light's short wavelength, it releases a higher amount of energy, which, over time, can cause serious long-term vision damage. Recent studies reveal that the effects of blue light exposure can result in an increased sensitivity to glare, reduced perception of contrast and color, a decrease in visual sharpness and, eventually it may lead to macular degeneration. According to *Bluelightexposed.com*, "Studies suggest that 60 percent of people spend more than 6 hours a day in front of a digital device."

Blue light isn't just emitted from electronic devices and energy-efficient fluorescent lighting. We are also exposed to it through natural sunlight. However, "in its natural form, your body uses blue light from the sun to regulate your natural sleep and wake cycles. [Natural] blue light also helps boost alertness, heighten reaction times, elevate moods, and increase the feeling of well-being" (*bluelightexposed.com*). When we are exposed to artificial forms of blue light, particularly at night, it can disrupt our sleep patterns, affect our appetite, and has been linked to an increased risk of certain cancers, heart disease, diabetes, and obesity.

Blue light's shorter wavelength causes it to "flicker more easily than [the] longer, weaker wavelengths" from the red end of the visible light spectrum (*bluelightexposed.com*). This flickering creates a glare which may be the cause behind the common complaints of eyestrain, headaches, and mental fatigue associated with spending extended periods of time in front of a screen. This prolonged exposure can cause retinal

> When my daughter told me she didn't need glasses anymore because of Ortho K offered by Dr. Roth, I could not believe it. Seeing that she is happy with it for over two years, I was wondering if this could work for me too. I was skeptical due to my age and my poor eyesight, but it works. I've used the Ortho K lenses for several years, and my quality of life has improved immensely. No more inconvenient glasses! Thank you Dr. Roth!
>
> ~ Doris (and Marcia)

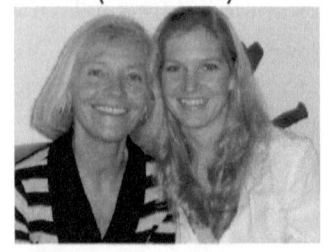

damage by bombarding the macula with high-energy light waves, which can lead to macular degeneration and ultimately, loss of central vision.

The macula is a small area of color-sensitive rods located in the center of the retina responsible for central vision (what we see directly in front of us). The macula or macular pigment acts in much the same way as the melanin in our skin, providing natural sun block. Prolonged exposure to blue light, as well as ultraviolet radiation (UVA and UVB rays), can reduce the density of the macular pigment, allowing more blue and ultraviolet light through, thus, damaging the retina.

According to a Harvard medical study "High Energy Visible (HEV) blue light has been identified for years as the most dangerous light for the retina. After chronic exposure, one can expect to see long-range growth in the number of macular degenerations, glaucoma, and retinal degenerative diseases." Another report published by the American Macular Degeneration Foundation states that "the blue rays of the spectrum seem to accelerate age-related macular degeneration more than any other rays in the spectrum." As discussed in Chapter Two, once vision is lost due to macular degeneration, there is no way to restore it.

Peripheral Retinal Defocus

Another major risk factor for the progression of myopia is myopia itself. People who are already myopic need to use some form of correction in order to regain clear vision. Traditionally, this correction came in the form of corrective lenses, either spectacles or contact lenses. Corrective lenses are still the most common method for correcting the refractive errors caused by myopia.

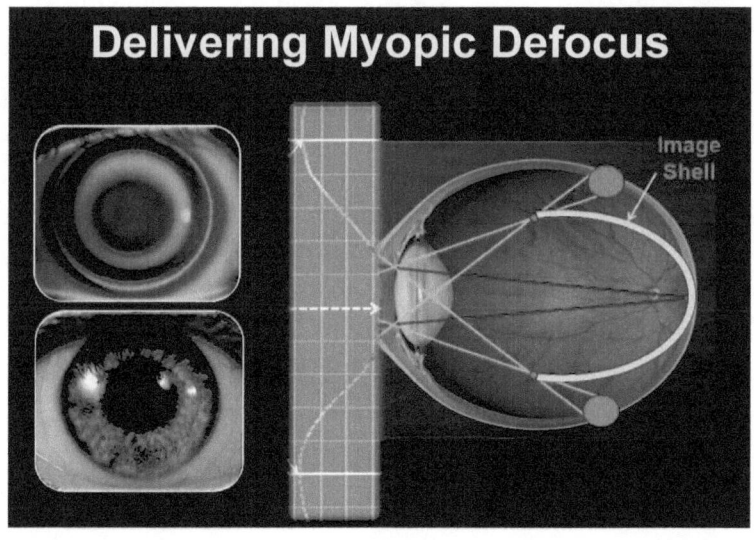

Most people never consider that their glasses or contacts could be harmful to their vision, when in fact their corrective lenses are more than likely making their myopia worse. It's hard for them to imagine that spectacles could do any harm when they don't even come into contact with their eyes. However, research has found that wearing corrective lenses, both glasses and contacts, allows for the negative progression of myopia. Since glasses and conventional contact lenses do not stop the progression of myopia, many patients who wear corrective lenses notice their myopia getting worse.

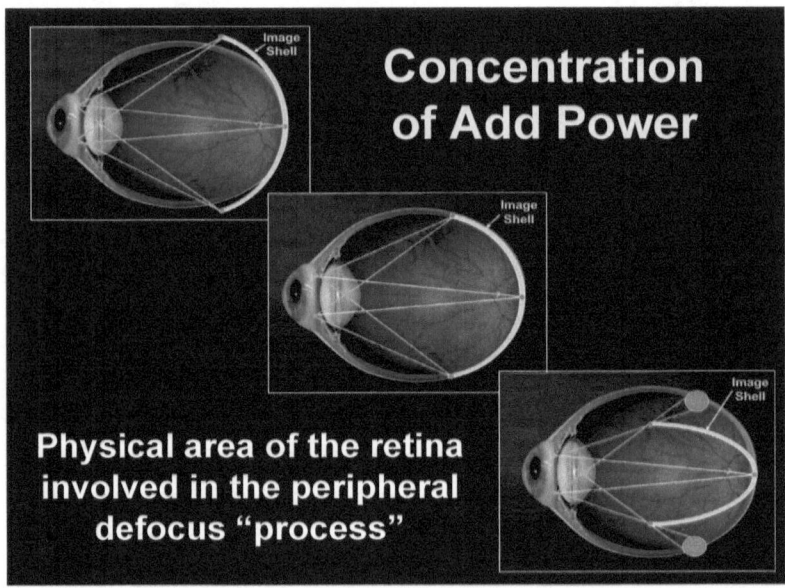

Myopiaprevention.org states that, "It is important to understand that the eye is not in focus across its entire retinal (back) surface at any one time." For myopic patients, particularly those who are used to wearing contact lenses, this may be a hard concept to grasp. They don't see the "side blur" in their peripheral vision that they usually have while wearing glasses, so they assume their vision must be in focus at all times while wearing contacts. However, just because their peripheral vision isn't blurry while wearing contacts, it doesn't mean their peripheral vision is in focus.

"The idea that the peripheral retina can be out of focus, either under- or over-focused, while the central straight ahead vision is in sharp focus is an important concept to understand" (myopiaprevention.org). The website also states that "Under-, full, and over-correction of central refractive error with single vision (soft contact lenses) caused a hyperopic shift in both central and peripheral refraction at all positions in the horizontal meridian." This means that by fitting a patient with single vision (as opposed to bifocal or multifocal) soft contact lenses, it creates a greater incidence of peripheral hyperopia. Hyperopia is the opposite of myopia. Thus, researchers have found that soft contact lenses cause the peripheral vision to become more farsighted. This change in the peripheral vision is one possible risk factor for the further progression of myopia.

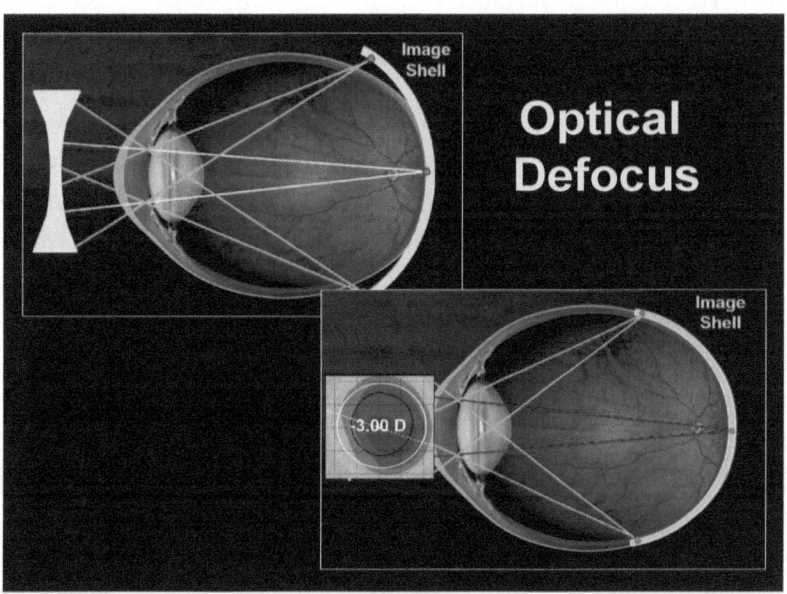

In January of 2010, a study was conducted, called the *Peripheral defocus with single-vision spectacle lenses in myopic children*. In the study, researchers suggested that "peripheral hyperopic defocus may play a role in the development and progression of myopia. We have shown that SVLs [single vision lenses] used to correct myopia can result in increased hyperopic defocus at the peripheral retina...this increase tends to escalate with increasing refractive error and eccentricity, especially in cases with moderate levels of myopia" (National Center for Biotechnology Information, a branch of the US National Library of Medicine website).

Peripheral retinal defocus is when light rays entering from the periphery do not focus on the back of the eye correctly. In peripheral hyperopic defocus, light doesn't come into focus within the eye at all (focusing beyond the retina). This refractive error can cause the eyes to increase in length, leading to myopia. As the length of the eyeball increases, the retina will begin to stretch in much the same way a balloon stretches as it is filled with more air. However, just as with a balloon, excessive stretching can cause a hole or tear in the retina to form, otherwise known as a retinal detachment.

Multiple studies have shown that using glasses or contacts to focus on objects that are straight in front of you may actually cause patients, particularly young patients whose eyes are still growing, to develop peripheral retinal defocus, making their myopia progress even more. While wearing glasses or contact lenses can correct current refractive errors and help central vision come into focus, they can cause myopia to become worse, increasing the risk of eye diseases and ultimately, blindness.

The use of glasses or contacts is not the only cause of peripheral retinal defocus. Even patients with normal sight can develop this condition. When we spend too much time indoors or live or work in congested urban areas, the peripheral vision can't focus on distant objects. The image in the center of the retina (our central vision) might be in focus, but the peripheral retina is blurred.

The good news is that if peripheral retinal defocus is caught early on and addressed, the deficits can be less severe later in life. By improving patients' peripheral focus, we can reduce their risk of developing eye diseases that can cause permanent loss of vision.

If glasses and contact lenses don't stop the progression of myopia, but can actually make it worse, you may be wondering what options you have left. Laser eye surgery can be risky, and just as with corrective lenses, it too doesn't stop the progression of myopia. The key is to stop thinking about correcting myopia, to stop simply applying temporary fixes, and start thinking about how you can control it.

CHAPTER SIX

A Case for Myopia Control Now

People have been wearing corrective lenses for literally hundreds of years. Corrective lenses have sufficiently enabled people with poor vision to see clearly again. Why then is there the need to focus on controlling myopia instead of simply correcting it as we have done for so long?

The current research on the prevalence of myopia proves that the condition is becoming a worldwide epidemic. This increase is due primarily to the introduction of computers and other electronic devices, as well as our increased time spent indoors. However, as discussed in the previous chapter, there are other factors involved. Evidence suggests that the use of traditional correction methods, such as glasses and contact lenses, won't stop the progression of myopia, and can actually make the condition worse.

For children, this may mean needing stronger and stronger prescriptions year after year. The more severe their myopia becomes, the more at risk they will become to eye diseases and other degenerative conditions such as retinal detachment and macular degeneration. Although glasses or contacts can improve vision in the short-term, they won't reduce the risk of your child going blind in the future. We can no longer focus on simply applying temporary fixes to aid our vision. The focus instead needs to be on controlling myopia so it can't progress any further.

Studies on myopia, as well as the negative impact of deteriorating vision, have shown that long-term vision health is dependent on myopia control. As discussed previously, progressive myopia has been proven to lead to an increased risk of retinal detachment and eye diseases, such as cataracts and glaucoma. These conditions, along with macular degeneration, all carry the risk of permanent vision loss.

As all of these conditions are risks of myopia, it goes without saying that controlling myopia, especially before it can become severe, is essential to preventing permanent vision loss. Once myopia reaches a certain point, there are little to no options for correction. According to the Royal National Institute for Blind People's (RNIB) website, severe or "high myopia is usually myopia over -6.00D." The *D* is an abbreviation for diopter, which is the unit of measurement for the refractive power of your eye's natural lens. As mentioned in Chapter Three, a prescription of -5.00D or higher increases the risk of myopic degeneration by 5,868 percent.

In addition to the eye-health risks associated with myopia, there are also significant social and personal costs. Hundreds of millions of people worldwide are dependent on corrective lenses in order to function on a daily basis. Many patients are unable to drive without their glasses or contacts. They cannot play sports, watch TV, or even get up during the night to go to the bathroom without their glasses. This dependency creates a personal cost, not only in regard to the expense of the corrective lenses but in the inconvenience they cause. For some patients, myopia has meant not getting the career or job they wanted or not being able to accomplish something as well as they had anticipated. Airline pilots, law-enforcement officers, and other occupations require clear vision to perform their tasks, and in many cases, simply correcting myopia with glasses or contacts is not enough.

The personal costs of myopia can include the aggravation associated with dependency. Losing a contact or breaking your glasses while you are away from home means having to change your plans. You might have to go home to get a spare pair of glasses or head to the eye doctor for new

> As I learned about these lenses through Dr. Reeder, I realized that they would fit perfectly with my occupation. Working as a marine mammal trainer at Sea World, I needed reliable vision both in and out of the water. I did not want to be concerned with losing a contact or getting something damaging in my eye or having impaired vision because of cloudy contacts. When I first started wearing the CRT lenses, I noticed that my vision seemed to have more depth. I find that my vision continues to have more contrast and I see things more vividly. Also, when I go for a run or ride my bicycle, a little dirt in my eye is no longer a painful hindrance as it gets trapped under a contact. Instead, it is just something I quickly blink away. There is no question in my mind that for an active individual, these lenses give you increased freedom.
>
> ~ Christine
> Patient of Dr. Sandler and Dr. Reeder

ones, assuming your doctor's office is even open at the time. Most eye-care clinics aren't open in the evenings or on weekends and holidays, yet glasses can break at any time. This inconvenience likely means having to depend on someone else to drive you around, or having to take time out of your day to get your glasses fixed or pick up new contacts. These problems may seem trivial to some, but they represent a personal cost, an unnecessary expense of time and energy. Unfortunately, this is a reality that those with corrective lenses have come to accept because they don't fully understand their options.

There are also social and financial costs to myopia. The corrective lens industry is based on consumption. Eyeglass and contact lens manufacturers profit from selling more glasses and contact lenses. Many of them also profit on the surgery, medical devices, and drugs needed once your eyes have deteriorated to a point of needing treatment beyond corrective lenses. You will find that most of the naysayers for myopia control are either involved with performing eye surgery, selling billions of dollars' worth of glasses or contact lenses, or selling the drugs needed once the damage is done. They have investors to satisfy. The safety, stabilization, and well-being of your child—and perhaps yourself—is not their number one priority.

Eye care is a business, a multi-billion dollar business. Add in the social and financial costs associated with the projected rate of increase in retinal detachments, macular degeneration, cataracts, glaucoma, and other serious eye diseases, and the numbers become astronomical. With the current state of health care, most people do not have adequate eye insurance. Many Americans don't have any eye insurance at all. This means the costs of annual eye exams, corrective lenses, or necessary eye surgery fall to the individual patients.

These expenses can lead to individuals not getting eye exams as frequently as they should, or to their not updating their prescriptions as often as they should. The recommendation is that glasses prescriptions be updated every two years, unless changes to the individual's vision are noticed prior to that, and contact prescriptions should be updated annually. Patients often wear contacts longer than they should to stretch out the cost and delay having to buy new ones. Glasses that are broken and taped back together continue to be worn because the individual isn't in a position to afford new frames.

Putting off eye exams, using outdated prescriptions, wearing broken glasses and old contact lenses all increase the risks of eye infections, worsening myopia, and ultimately, eye disease. I have witnessed people with eye diseases put off treatment or even the initial exam because they were trying to avoid the costs associated with getting adequate care. Some of these people, who then suffered a retinal detachment, are now permanently blind because they waited too long to go to the eye doctor. Some elderly patients with cataracts waited until they literally couldn't see any more before having the surgery. As an eye doctor, these are just some of the many personal and social costs of myopia that I see on a regular basis.

So, why is myopia control so important now when myopia has been a problem for centuries? There are two answers to that question. First, the prevalence of myopia is higher now than ever before and constantly increasing. The Koffler Vision Group's website states that "In just the last generation, the rate of myopia has increased in the US by 65 percent." Also, the lack of time spent outside and the dramatic increase in time spent on electronic devices, along with the effects of the blue light exposure associated with that increased use, has changed eye health for entire societies. As explained earlier in this book, we are now facing a myopia epidemic that will continue to grow if myopia control is not embraced.

The second answer to that question is that we now have the ability to control myopia as never before. In addition to some simple changes you can make in your everyday life that can help slow the progression of myopia, which will be discussed in the following chapter, there are new and emerging options available that can safely and effectively stop the progression of myopia and give patients clear vision. Some of these options have been around for decades, but it is only recently that we have the research to support their safety and effectiveness.

One of these options, and the subject of this book, is orthokeratology (awr-thoh-ker-*uh*-**tol**-*uh*-jee). *Dictionary.com* defines orthokeratology as "a technique for correcting refractive errors in vision by changing the shape of the cornea with the temporary use of progressively flatter hard contact lenses." Called Ortho-K for short, this technique has the potential to halt the ongoing progression of myopia.

Despite the long-term benefits and effectiveness of Ortho-K, there are still some people, even within the eye-health community, who do not recognize it as a viable option for controlling myopia. However, there have been multiple studies conducted in different countries examining its effectiveness. These studies, which will be discussed in detail later in this book, demonstrate the benefits of orthokeratology on significantly slowing and even stopping the progression of myopia.

Some have argued that myopia can be corrected with laser eye surgery, which eliminates the need for daily corrective lenses and has a high success rate. As discussed previously, laser eye surgery essentially does nothing in regard to controlling myopia. Laser surgery can correct your current myopia; however, your eye will continue to stretch as you age, which means that over time, the positive impact of the surgery will be lost. Once this happens, your options for correcting your vision will be limited due to the thinning of the cornea from both the myopia and the laser surgery.

In addition to orthokeratology, there are other options available for myopia control, which will be examined in in the following chapter.

> I recently finished the Gentle Molding Therapy (Ortho-k) with Dr. Roth and I could not be more thrilled with the results! I don't have to wear contacts during the day anymore. I can finally exercise and go swimming without having to worry about my contacts. I can even take a spontaneous nap during the day without having to worry about first removing my contact lenses. When I recently renewed my driver's license and they asked whether I need glasses or contact lenses to drive, I could finally say no! I'm so grateful for finding Dr. Roth and making the decision to try the therapy. It has changed my life.
>
> Marcia

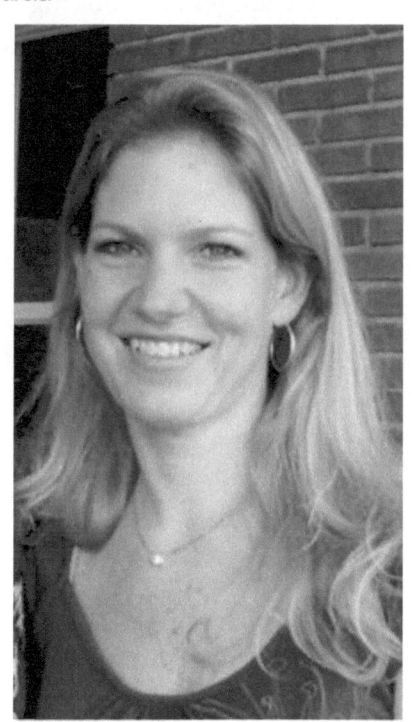

Of these options, Ortho-K is arguably the most effective, with the longest-lasting benefits. Most patients with myopia are good candidates for Ortho-K. Only a small percentage of patients would not benefit from this option due to the condition of their eyes, or due to a previous attempt at other refractive therapies and they found them to be unsuccessful in correcting their current myopia.

The bottom line is that the prevalence of myopia is exploding in many developed countries. Current projections suggest that over thirty-five million Americans will be myopic by the year 2030, with nearly forty-five million by the year 2050. As the younger generations continue to age, the prevalence of myopia, eye diseases, and retinal detachment will only increase. Clearly, there is a need for myopia control now.

Educating the public on the causes and complications of myopia can increase efforts to prevent the spread of this condition. However, reeducating an entire society (if not the entire world) and convincing them to change their daily habits is a complicated and challenging endeavor. By educating people on the benefits and options for controlling myopia and lessening our social dependence on glasses and daytime contacts, we are taking a step in the right direction. Simply making a few lifestyle changes and looking into alternative options, you can take charge of your child's myopia (and maybe your own) and stop it in its tracks.

CHAPTER SEVEN

Options for Myopia Control

The risks associated with myopia, which were discussed in previous chapters, are well-established concerns. Understanding them, along with the reasons for the dramatic increase in myopia prevalence, has led more and more researchers to study options for controlling this devastating condition instead of simply correcting it.

Similar to studies conducted regarding the prevalence of myopia, the majority of the studies done on myopia control has been conducted in developed countries, such as the United States, New Zealand, Australia, China, Japan, and Taiwan, to name a few. Several different options for myopia control have been explored so far, but each option comes with its own list of benefits and potential complications to consider.

While myopia control is relevant and important for both adults and children, much of the research conducted thus far has focused on children. This is due to the fact that myopia can still be prevented if measures are taken before the condition begins to develop. In myopic patients of younger ages, the condition can be slowed or even halted, meaning it won't progress any further. However, once myopia develops, it cannot be reversed.

While nearly all of the vision-correction methods available provide temporary relief from poor vision, they do not change or eliminate the presence of myopia. Therefore, many doctors are now focusing on control methods that will actually slow or stop the progression of myopia in children entirely, so it does not progress to a point of causing retinal detachment, serious eye diseases, or eventual blindness when they become adults.

As discussed previously, research has found that the dramatic increase in the prevalence of myopia is related to the significant rise in near work in recent years.

Kids are spending more time inside, reading, studying, watching television, and using electronic devices. Our eyes are not designed for such concentrated focus on near work, especially for long periods of time. Therefore, the options for myopia control are separated into two categories. The first category consists of ways to help prevent myopia to begin with, and the second consists of ways for controlling the progression of this degenerative condition. It is never too late to start working toward controlling your myopia.

For children, it is important to establish good habits while they are still young, as these habits will stay with them as they age. These good habits include regularly spending time outside. The Koffler Vision Group website recommends that you "make sure your kids include going outside for walks, trips to the park, or playing outdoor sports as part of their daily routine." Many doctors believe that spending more than two hours outside every day is the turning point for slowing the progression of myopia. The combination of natural light exposure and relying on distance vision are key benefits to being outdoors.

Children should also maintain a safe distance while reading, watching television, and using electronic devices. Equally important is to avoid long stretches of time focusing on near work without a break. Obviously, it is impossible for kids to completely avoid using electronic devices as the use of computers and tablets in the classroom continues to increase. However, they can avoid using them for hours a day without taking breaks.

Most schools are now relying more and more on electronic devices, so it is important that teachers, as well as parents, understand the need for visual breaks. Teachers should allocate time for students to take small breaks from computers or tablets, as well as allowing them breaks while reading and watching the smart boards or projection screens used in the classroom. This can be as simple as having students look away from their books or screens for a period of time.

I encourage my patients to follow the 20-20-20 rule. When using an electronic device, the child should look away from the screen every twenty minutes and focus on something that is at least twenty feet away for at least twenty seconds. Doing this will give the eyes a break from working so hard to focus on the short distance. This rule can be helpful to both children and adults. While the 20-20-20 rule may help slow the progression of myopia, the most ideal situation would be to limit screen time altogether. The light emitted from modern device screens is just as damaging to our eyes, if not more so, as the distance at which they are viewed. However, due to educational needs and school requirements, limiting overall screen time may be unrealistic.

Our son, Kaleb, who was 10 at the time, went for his annual medical exam, and it was noted that his eye vision was 20/70. Furthermore, he tells us that he has been unable to see the board at school and how it was affecting his sports, which was news to us. We were referred to Dr. Roth by a friend who just obtained GMT (Ortho K) for their son and had great results. We made the consult appointment and decided to go this route. After a day of sleeping in the contacts, we returned to Dr. Roth for his follow up. His vision parameters had stabilized and he was seeing 20/20. We returned the 2nd day and his vision was 20/15.

We recently completed a year of using GMT and Kaleb is still seeing 20/15 and his vision parameters (contact power) has stayed the same.

To say the least, we have been very pleased and would highly recommend Dr. Roth and GMT to anyone. Our son has been able to see things more clear, sharp and is pleased regarding the sport he plays and the vision he has obtained. This had definitely helped his performance in the classroom and on the field.

We, as his parents, couldn't be any more happier with the results. Thank you Dr. Roth and we look forward to continued success!!!!

Some may argue that in a classroom setting, it is impossible for all students to focus on something more than twenty feet away. Only those seated next to the windows are able to do so. While following the 20-20-20 rule may be difficult depending on the structure and size of the classroom, it is important to realize that this rule can still help preserve good vision. Myopia is a condition that should be considered just as important as any other health issue. If a teacher were told that all she had to do to save her students from losing their vision as adults was to let them look out the window periodically throughout the day, that teacher would no doubt feel compelled to comply. It is as simple as that.

The real problem is that not enough people realize the seriousness of this situation. Long periods of time spent focusing on electronic devices is damaging our children's vision at an accelerated rate.

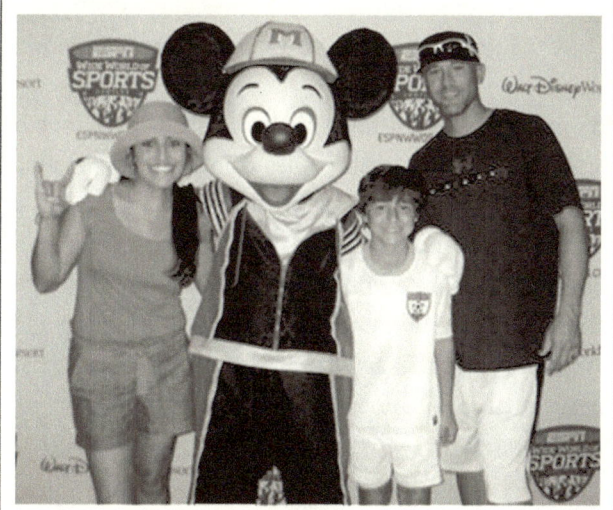

In addition to the 20-20-20 rule, another way to help decrease the risk of damage to your eyes is by spending time outside. Not sitting outside reading a book or using an electronic device, but actually doing something that forces you to focus on objects at long distances. This can be walking, playing, or just watching the world go by. Allowing your eyes to focus on distant objects strengthens their natural abilities. Think about this another way. When people are sedentary for a long period of time, their muscles weaken. The longer the periods of time become, the greater their muscle weakness, until it impacts their ability to move. That is why it is so important for people to stay active. The same idea applies to the eyes. If you don't force them to focus at long distances regularly, they can lose their ability to do so, and they can become myopic.

Being outside also exposes the eyes to natural light, as opposed to the harsh light of overhead fixtures or the blue light emitted from digital screens and energy-efficient fluorescent lighting. Believed to be a huge contributing factor to the increase in eye problems, blue light is the most dangerous form of light for the eyes, according to recent studies. Natural light is the most beneficial for children and adults. Children should be outside for a minimum of twelve to fourteen hours per week. Recent research strongly suggests that natural sunlight is not only beneficial, but the lack of it can actually increase the risk of myopia.

The prevalence of myopia in Asian countries has been so significant that in some areas, they are redesigning schools to allow for more time under natural light conditions. They are incorporating the outdoor into classrooms by installing glass walls and ceilings. A small study in Taiwan examined the prevalence of myopia among students in one of these glass classrooms versus students in a traditional classroom. Of the students in the glass classroom, only 8 percent developed myopia, while 18 percent of the students in the traditional classroom developed the condition.

Although the research into natural light and its effect on the prevalence of myopia has been ongoing for several years, it is still in its infancy. Researchers in several parts of the world are working to determine the ideal amount of sunlight developing eyes need, as well as other factors such as the degree of sunlight. For example, is midday sunlight more beneficial than early morning or late afternoon sunlight? Is the benefit still there if the child is wearing UV protective sunglasses? Researchers in Australia are looking into the correlation between the amount of time spent outdoors, the prevalence of myopia, and the risk of sun damage to the eyes. This particular group of researchers is trying to determine whether the risk of sun damage outweighs the benefits of reducing the risk of myopia.

Despite the fact that there is still a lot to learn regarding the risks and benefits of natural light, the general consensus among researchers is that natural light has a significantly positive impact on reducing the risk of myopia in children.

Other good habits to instill in children include holding their book or electronic device at least eight inches away from their face and below eye level. Kids will often lie on their side with their book or electronic device flat on the floor. This causes them to focus out of the corner of their eyes in order to see. This is very bad for the eyes as it can add to the deterioration of their vision. When reading, kids should be sitting with the book or electronic device in front of them, either on a table or in their lap.

These tips apply to adults as well. According to recent research, nine out of ten adults spend more than two hours a day on a digital device. Six out of ten adults spend more than five hours a day on a digital device. Furthermore, one out of three adults born between 1965 and 1980 spend nine or more hours a day on a digital device, mainly due to their jobs. Similar to children in school, it is often difficult for adults to not spend prolonged periods of time on electronic devices. However, adults can also practice the 20-20-20 rule.

Three factors that contribute to digital eyestrain are the close to mid-range distance between the eyes and the screen, the decrease in blinking, and the prolonged exposure to blue light emitted from modern digital screens. The majority of people hold their electronic devices dangerously close to their eyes. They do so for many reasons. First, trying to focus on small words and blurry images is difficult, so people tend to bring the device closer to their eyes in order to focus more clearly. The second common reason is for comfort. Many people are on their electronic devices while lying down or lounging in a chair. These positions naturally cause people to hold their devices closer to their face to ease neck strain or stiffness in their backs or shoulders.

Prolonged use of digital devices naturally leads to decreased blinking. Most people don't even realize they are blinking less until they finally look away and notice the discomfort in their eyes or have trouble readjusting their vision to their surroundings. Blinking is an important function for overall eye health. Each time you blink, a salty solution from your tear ducts sweeps over the eye's surface. This acts as a moisturizer for the eye, and washes away dust particles and protein deposits that can settle on the surface of the eye.

Digital eyestrain can cause eyes to feel dry, itchy, or burning. If you wear contacts, digital eyestrain can make them feel irritating. It can also negatively impact tear production, causing dry eye disease. The negative effects of digital eyestrain are becoming significantly more prevalent as more adults are dependent on electronic devices and not doing anything to protect their vision. Research on the long-term effects of digital eyestrain is still ongoing.

In addition to the daily habit changes already discussed, you can also invest in computer eyewear. These are specially-designed glasses that block the blue light emitted from digital screens from entering our eyes. Wearing computer eyewear does not impact the quality of your vision when looking at electronic devices, and consistently wearing them can decrease the risk of digital eyestrain. These glasses may be very helpful for those who need to work at a computer all day. Computer glasses may also be helpful for children.

Preventing damage to your eyes is essential for everyone, regardless of age or current eye health. However, once you have myopia, it is important to understand your options for controlling your condition. The risks are serious ones that can lead to eye surgeries and the possibility of permanent vision loss. For this reason, controlling myopia instead of allowing it to progress is an important endeavor. Yet, myopia control is not widely practiced in most areas. The focus is still on the treatment of myopia through the use of corrective lenses, with little to no consideration of preventing or slowing the condition.

Making these simple lifestyle changes can go a long way to slowing myopia in already myopic patients or preventing it in those who have not yet developed

> I have worn glasses/contacts all my life since the age of five. To finally be able to not have to wear anything on my face or in my eyes for most of the day is wonderful freedom. Dr. Roth's patience and exceptional professional knowledge was such an asset in helping me to make the choice towards having the procedure (GMT Gentle Molding Therapy) done. I am now recommending to others to have the procedure (GMT) instead of "Laser" surgery.
>
> Angela

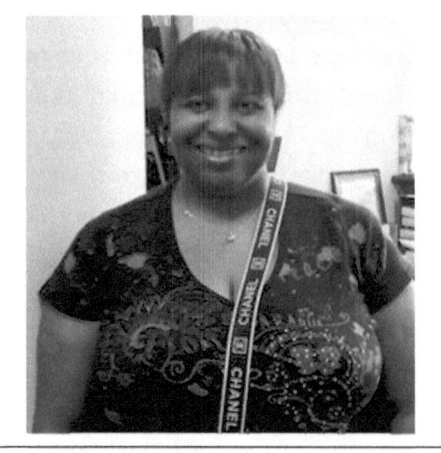

the condition. There are also several recognized treatment options that can slow the progression of myopia. These include atropine drops, soft multifocal contact lenses, or orthokeratology lenses. Recent research supports the use and effectiveness of each of these methods to slow or stop the progression of myopia. Which method you choose will depend strongly on the severity of your myopia, your age, and which options your eye doctor may offer.

Atropine Drops

Atropine drops are a topical medicine used to dilate the pupil and temporarily cause the eyes' focusing mechanism to relax. These drops are commonly used to treat eye pain caused by some forms of uveitis or eye inflammation. Atropine drops were initially considered for myopia control due to the research that cited focusing fatigue as a possible cause of nearsightedness in children.

The drops are placed in the eyes at night before going to bed. They dilate the eyes for several hours, thus forcing the eye muscles to relax. This is believed to give the eyes an opportunity to rest and recover, slowing the elongation of the axial of the eyeball, which leads to worsening myopia. Some eye doctors use atropine drops in very young patients who are already demonstrating worsening myopia but are too young to wear corrective lenses.

Between 1989 and 2010, four independent studies were conducted to determine the effectiveness of atropine drops in slowing the progression of myopia. These studies found, on average, an 81 percent reduction in myopia progression in children while using the drops. Some research has suggested that the effectiveness of atropine drops is not ongoing, with the most significant reduction only seen in the first year of use. However, follow-up studies have also found that the short-term use of atropine drops maintained a lasting effect. One study tested children two years after discontinuing the atropine drops. They showed more sustained control over their myopia.

While atropine drops have demonstrated positive results in controlling myopia, many doctors are hesitant to use them due to the potential complications. Atropine drops may cause discomfort in the eyes and light sensitivity. They have also been found to cause near vision to get blurry. While the patient's far vision is improved, they may need bifocals for near work. Additionally, some doctors argue that there is not enough research on the potential long-term complications of using atropine drops for children.

Multifocal Soft Contact Lenses (MSCLs)

Another option in myopia control is the use of multifocal soft contact lenses. Multifocal contact lenses are designed to have different prescription strengths in different zones of the lens (multiple focal points). Several studies have demonstrated their effectiveness in reducing the progression of myopia. The results of a six-month study in 2010, involving 115 children between the ages of seven and fourteen revealed that the children wearing the MSCLs had 54 percent less progression than the children wearing glasses. A similar study conducted in 2011 in New Zealand showed a 30 percent difference in the reduction of myopia progression. Still, a third study conducted in the United States in 2013 reported that the group of children wearing multifocal contact lenses showed 50 percent less myopia progression than the control group, all of whom wore regular contact lenses.

While the results of these three studies varied in regard to the percentage difference in reduction, they all demonstrated a clear change in the vision of the children tested. These studies prove that multifocal soft contact lenses work to reduce the progression of myopia. How well they work is still being determined through ongoing research, but they are a clear option for patients interested in myopia control. The potential complications of using multifocal soft contact lenses are no different than those associated with wearing regular contact lenses. All contact lenses require proper hygiene and care. They may cause irritation, and there is a risk of infection if they are not properly cleaned and stored.

Orthokeratology

Orthokeratology, which is the focus of this book, is the use of overnight hard contact lenses designed to reshape the cornea. Ortho-K lenses may also be referred to as corneal reshaping lenses or corneal refractive therapy (CRT). These lenses are gas-permeable contact lenses that are specially designed to temporarily "fix" nearsightedness. Ortho-K lenses are worn by the patient only at night while they are sleeping, allowing them freedom from corrective lenses during the day.

The specially-shaped lenses work by gently reshaping the cornea, which is the clear, domed surface of your eye. Properly shaping the cornea allows light entering the eye to bend (refract) correctly, restoring perfect or near-perfect vision. Due to the cornea's fluid nature, the effects of the reshaping will only last throughout the day, so the lenses need to be worn every night to maintain clear vision. Research has shown that vision improves approximately 50 percent each night the lenses are worn, so it may take a couple of days of wearing them to achieve perfect vision.

The risks associated with Ortho-K lenses are no different than the risks involved with regular contact lenses. The same care in properly cleaning, handling, and storing the lenses should be taken. Not doing so can lead to eye infections such as microbial keratitis. As mentioned, because the visual benefits of Ortho-K lenses are temporary, there are no long-term side effects on the eye or to the vision.

Ortho-K lenses are used to immediately correct vision in both children and adults. However, research has shown that they are also effective in myopia control. Multiple studies have been conducted measuring the progression of myopia in children using Ortho-K lenses as opposed to traditional glasses or contacts. In nearly every study, the progression of myopia was significantly less in the children wearing Ortho-K lenses. These studies will be explored further in Chapter Eight.

Some patients may consider corrective surgery as a way to control their myopia. While laser surgeries such as LASIK, have become increasingly popular in recent years due to improvements to the technology, laser eye surgery does not stop the progression of myopia. Therefore, it is not an effective method for myopia control.

Myopia control is not a new endeavor. However, relative to the long history of the eyeglass industry, it is a fairly recent concept. The number of eye doctors providing myopia control options is quickly growing as more and more realize the need for myopia control now. Researchers are also continuing to look for better, more viable options. When considering your options, it is important to talk to your eye doctor about what methods for myopia control he or she provides. Even with all the available options out there, we believe that orthokeratology is the gold standard in myopia control.

CHAPTER EIGHT

The Gold Standard

As optometrists, we can offer various options of myopia control. We understand the value of each method and the importance of determining which option is best suited for each of our patients. Hundreds of patients come through my practice every week. I work with patients as young as kindergarten and all the way up through advanced adulthood. I have a great team of colleagues who work with me, and are all committed to myopia control and helping our patients preserve their eye health.

One of the goals I have for my practice is to educate people regarding the risks associated with myopia. As a society, wearing corrective lenses has become the standard for dealing with this condition. It is not uncommon nowadays to see children in first and second grade already wearing glasses, and it is even worse in other parts of the world, particularly in Asia.

The increase in myopia prevalence in many Asian countries, such as China, is frightening. There are some areas with an 80 to 90 percent prevalence. This means the vast majority of the population in those areas is now myopic and dependent on corrective lenses or some other form of myopic correction. This is why much of the early research and trials done on overnight corneal reshaping lenses were conducted in Asian countries. They recognized that the situation was escalating and knew something had to be done to increase the success of myopia-control methods.

It is only in recent years that more countries have recognized the need for further research into the causes and possible solutions of myopia. Developed countries are all seeing a dramatic increase in myopia prevalence, and many countries, including the United States, Australia, and Spain, have started conducting myopia-control research. However, the general public is still generally unaware of the risks associated with this progressive condition.

I do not promote myopia control to my patients as a means of simply avoiding glasses or contacts. While that is a clear benefit to controlling myopia, my true concern is for the long-term vision health of my patients. The growing number of children experiencing severe myopia at younger and younger ages is very disconcerting. The eyes of most people do not stabilize until they are in their early twenties. If kids are now developing myopia as young as kindergarten, the condition of their eyes will be severe by the time they reach maturity. Severe myopia dramatically increases the risk of developing eye diseases like glaucoma and macular degeneration, as well as retinal tearing or detachment. Thus, by the time these kids grow into adulthood, there is going to be an epidemic of eye diseases and retinal detachments. The social and financial burden on our society will be extreme.

I first became interested in the specifics of myopia control after witnessing two family members experience retinal detachments. This is a devastating experience for anyone. Even if it is caught quickly, it still means months of uncomfortable treatments, possible surgery, and lengthy recovery time. That is the best-case scenario. If it is not caught in time, it could mean permanent vision loss. Many people do not seek immediate help when experiencing a retinal detachment because they are unaware of the warning signs. Retinal detachments are not painful due to the lack of pain receptors in the eye, so people tend to ignore the symptoms.

An individual's risk of retinal detachment is significantly increased when the patient has severe myopia (-5.00D or higher). The elongation of the eyeball puts too much stress on the retina, which leads to tearing, holes, and eventually partial or full detachment, which can result in permanent vision loss. Looking into the future, if nothing is done to educate the general public regarding the need for myopia control now, blindness may become as common as corrective lenses are today.

The need for services aimed at helping people with vision loss will explode. Today, retinal detachment is still relatively uncommon. You may know of someone who has experienced it, but it isn't common enough that you likely know of multiple people who have experienced it. Yet. I say *yet* because this will change. As early as the next decade, retinal detachment will become commonplace unless something is done to control the increasing prevalence and severity of myopia.

The same will happen with ocular diseases. Cataracts, glaucoma, and macular degeneration are still considered age-related eye diseases. The general public does not understand the connection between the development of these diseases and myopia. As the current generation of corrective-lens-dependent people age, there will be an explosion in the number of patients developing ocular diseases. The ages at which these patients are diagnosed will also decrease, and we will start to see younger and younger adults with eye diseases once thought to occur only in the elderly.

More outdoor time is highly valuable to everyone, regardless of age or whether or not they are myopic. Sufficient outdoor time has been proven to not only prevent the development of myopia, but to slow the progression of it. However, between work and school commitments, many people see increasing their outdoor time as unrealistic. I work to educate these patients on the value of protecting their vision now, so they can reap the benefits later. Since I can only make recommendations, it has to be up to the patients to take an active role in their own eye health.

The overall decrease in time spent outdoors is also a societal problem. In some Asian countries, where myopia is recognized as a severe societal concern, there are special classrooms

> I'd like to thank Dr. David Roth for helping me achieve what I thought could only be possible with Lasik, which I have always had reservations about and have long sought an alternative for. I had heard about Ortho-K before and had shoved it aside since I felt that my near-sightedness was likely too bad to fix; plus I had never worn contacts. After coming across this procedure again in the Herald article, however, I thought there might be something to it and decided to give it a shot. The fact that since the third day of going through the process I have had 20/20 vision or near it on most days and have not used my glasses once still feels incredible to say the least; my only regret now is that I wish I would have done this much sooner. If there would have been more optometrists like Dr. Roth touting this therapy back when I first needed to start wearing glasses I'm sure my eyesight wouldn't have degraded so much since I would've opted for that which would lessen the progression of my condition. Nonetheless, I am grateful that he is one of those practicing it and helping it get the publicity it deserves.
>
> Michael
>
>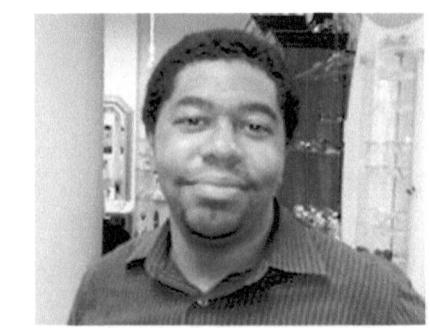

being built with glass walls and ceilings so children can attend school while still getting the benefits of natural lighting and forced use of their distance vision.

In my practice, I utilize and promote all necessary forms of myopia control, whatever is best suited to the individual patient. For example, some patients are simply too young to be fitted with contacts. For these patients, I encourage lots of outdoor time and atropine drops. Depending on the severity of their myopia, I may recommend multifocal soft contacts. This option provides more long-term results than the drops, and it may be well-suited for patients not helped by orthokeratology.

Although there are pros and cons to each method of myopia control, in my professional opinion, orthokeratology is the gold standard. Unless I'm working with a patient who cannot use Ortho-K lenses, or the patient is in strict opposition to using them for one reason or another, it is my standard recommendation.

Ortho-K lenses have been proven through numerous studies to not only correct current vision problems but to actually slow down and stop the progression of myopia. With the exception of one study that I know of, every study conducted to examine the progression of myopia using Ortho-K lenses as opposed to using other methods demonstrates the advantages of Ortho-K. This includes studies done to compare Ortho-K lenses to glasses, soft contacts, a control group wearing nothing, and other myopia correction methods.

In addition to the clear evidence presented in these studies, I've been able to witness its effectiveness firsthand with my own patients. My success rate in slowing the progression of their myopia with Ortho-K lenses is extremely high. Ortho-K is making a difference in the lives of my patients, reducing their risk to eye diseases and retinal detachment, and preserving the health of their eyes for the long-term.

Many of my patients have asked me why I think Ortho-K isn't more mainstream and why more people don't know about this option for controlling myopia. On an even more basic level, they are curious as to why more people don't understand the dangers of not getting their myopia under control. My answer to these questions is simple. The problem has to do with knowledge. There is an overwhelming lack of education, not only in our country, but around the world. People need to be better informed in order to make accurate decisions regarding the health of their eyes and their children's eyes.

When a belief has been held by a culture for generations, people are slow to change, even when faced with overwhelming evidence. The same is true for the belief that corrective lenses are the answer to myopia. People are slow to open up their minds to new information. Anytime an alternative treatment is offered, there is going to be skepticism, at least initially. However, instead of viewing Ortho-K as a type of alternative medicine, you should view it as a revolutionary treatment. It should be seen as a breakthrough in eye health because that is exactly what it is.

Ortho-K offers the first reasonable and proven-effective method to slow the progression of myopia. It has the potential to actually control the associated loss of vision due to severe myopia for the first time in the history of the eye-care industry. The same cannot be said for corrective lenses or laser eye surgery. Controlling the progression of myopia instead of applying quick fixes is really the key difference in long-term vision health, and it is what makes Ortho-K the gold standard in myopia control.

My goal in being a part of this book is to use it as a vehicle to educate others. While many people think that myopia control is a relatively new concept, since they have never heard about it before, the idea itself has actually been around for generations. Even the technology behind Ortho-K has been around for a long time. The current form of orthokeratology was developed over forty years, as doctors and researchers tested and tried different approaches to figure out what worked.

I want all parents to know they have options in protecting their children's eye health. They don't have to stand by, helpless, and watch their children's eyes get progressively worse year after year as they become increasingly dependent on corrective lenses. They don't have to worry about their children developing a devastating eye disease and risk permanent loss of their vision as they grow up.

Likewise, I want every adult who has been living with myopia to know there are options to regain control of their vision. They don't have to deal with the hassle and inconvenience of corrective lenses for the rest of their lives. They don't have to undergo a risky surgery in the hope that it may correct their vision, if only temporarily.

People need to learn the risks associated with myopia, as well as strategies to prevent and ways to control it. They need to be educated about Ortho-K and the possibilities it presents for most patients living with myopia. When compared to corrective lenses and laser surgery, the benefits of Ortho-K are overwhelming.

As an eye doctor, I could talk for hours about the benefits of orthokeratology and how it has helped countless patients. However, I think is much more effective to let some of my patients speak for themselves about their own experiences and the benefits they received from Ortho-K. I get the opportunity to work with a diverse group of patients, and I am proud and honored when they come back to thank us for everything we have given them. Ortho-K has truly helped them live a better life.

CHAPTER NINE

Orthokeratology
Stuart Grant, O.D.

Orthokeratology was a term coined by my partner, Charles May, O.D., and me back in the 1950s when we first discovered the concept of reshaping the cornea to temporarily correct vision. In an article entitled *Orthokeratology: Reshaping Corneas, Redefining Ideas*, Adrienne McQueen, NCLC, explains that "when the word is broken down into its Greek origins, *orthokeratology* can be defined as 'the science of straight corneas.'" As the name implies, we use the methods and technology developed over the last five decades to safely improve and correct our patients' vision and ultimately stop the progression of myopia.

However, the theory behind orthokeratology may date back even farther. There is a legend from ancient China that tells of a man who had gone to "sleep with his face resting on his forearm. When he awoke, he noticed that his normally blurred vision was suddenly clear. He suspected that the pressure he'd put on his eyes was the reason, and soon physicians were telling their myopic patients to go to bed with sandbags on their eyelids. The treatment is still prescribed in China" (*Los Angeles Magazine*, January 2004). We know today that it was the pressure of his forearm gently reshaping his corneas that had temporarily cleared his blurred vision.

During the 1950s, Dr. May and I, who were working out of the same optometry office at the time, had discovered the benefits of orthokeratology quite by accident. Hard contact lenses made of polymethylmethacrylate (PMMA), the first alternative to spectacles, had just become available. Before that, the only option patients had for correcting their vision was glasses, which had been around in one form or another since the thirteenth century.

After we began fitting patients with these new lenses, we had some of them coming back in for check-ups and telling us they were able to see better even when they weren't wearing their contacts. They'd tell me they'd get halfway to work in the morning and realize they hadn't put their lenses in, which made no sense whatsoever. It was hard to believe at first, but when we checked their eyes, we discovered that indeed, their vision had improved.

The contacts had flattened the cornea and changed its curvature. By reducing the overall axial length of the eyeball through flattening the cornea and by changing the cornea's curvature, the angle at which light entered the eye was also changed, causing it to reflect more correctly on the retina. We speculated that if the cornea could be unintentional reshaped, perhaps it could be reshaped intentionally in a controlled manner. We began to research what the cornea could tolerate, and started looking at treating the condition of myopia instead of just coping with it.

Orthokeratology lenses are designed to apply gentle pressure to the cornea to create a desired corneal shape. By reshaping the cornea, light that enters the eye is refracted correctly (meaning the light focuses directly on the retina instead of in front of it), allowing for clearer distance vision. When forced to focus for long periods of time, especially on up-close objects, the eye can begin to stretch and lengthen, causing myopia. By reducing this lengthening, we can effectively slow down the progression of myopia. "With record numbers of young people becoming more nearsighted every year, orthokeratology's greatest advantage lies in its potential to forestall myopia, not just heal it on a daily basis" (*Los Angeles Magazine,* January 2004).

Around the same time, there were many other doctors also experimenting with the use of rigid contacts to reshape the cornea, each of them contributing to the development of this technology in different ways. Through our own research, Dr. May and I developed a specific method that used a series of relatively large, flat lenses with larger optic zone diameters (OZDs) than standard lenses. The larger diameter allowed for better centering of the lens on the cornea. "The most important factor for a successful fit is good lens centration. To safely produce the maximum reduction of myopia and astigmatism, the flattest possible fit that centers well is desired" (Adrienne McQueen, *Orthokeratology: Reshaping Corneas, Redefining Ideas*).

Similar to dental retainers, each lens would flatten the cornea a small amount until we finally achieved the desired result, a process that sometimes took months or years back then. We found that making small changes to the cornea by using progressively more precise lenses produced safer and more effective results for our patients. Today, the same results can be achieved much quicker because of the advancements in lens materials and manufacturing equipment.

Over the years, we researched different materials for use in our lenses, not only in the pursuit of better results but to increase patient comfort as well. We found that lenses made with certain materials were more gas-permeable. Allowing more oxygen to pass through the lens meant improved comfort for our patients and improved overall eye health, reducing the risks of diseases like dry eye and glaucoma. "These materials were far more physiologically compatible to the cornea... Also, because of the enhanced permeability they provided, larger diameter gas-permeable Ortho-K lenses could be used" (Adrienne McQueen, *Orthokeratology: Reshaping Corneas, Redefining Ideas*).

There have also been advances in the equipment used to produce the lenses in recent years. We can now scan and precisely map the topography of each individual patient's cornea, using reverse geometry to engineer custom lenses. There are computerized lathes that can produce the custom lenses quickly and accurately, eliminating the risks of the one-size-fits-all kits of some corneal reshaping methods. Using reverse geometry to construct the lenses also allowed us to keep them centered on the cornea, increasing the lens' effectiveness in flattening and shortening the cornea.

> I've been wearing glasses and regular day tie contact lenses for over 10 years. They would always inhibit my ability to enjoy the beach, the pool or sports while growing up. Unfortunately, I was too you and hesitant for Lasik, so when I heard about Ortho k and Dr. Roth, I knew I had to try it. I was fitted for my retainers right before the start of my first year of college and immediately I could tell Ortho k would be life changing. Having used Ortho K for just over a year now, I can say with all confidence that the retainers are extremely easy to use and not having to use glasses or contacts during the day has been an amazing gift. I can finally enjoy my days without the use of inhibiting day-time contacts. Thank you Dr. Roth!
>
> Alesandro

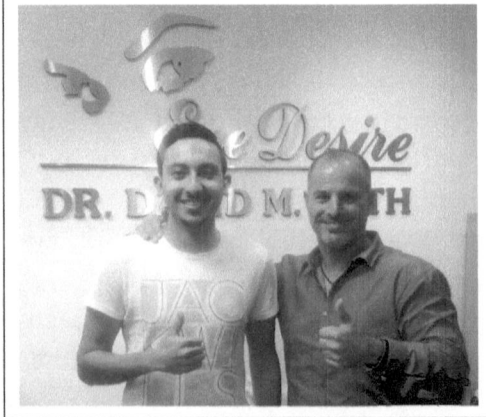

With myopia, the axial length of the eyeball can increase as the cornea becomes more steeply curved. Ortho-K lenses keep the cornea from continuing to protrude through the use of a rigid contact. The contact lens creates a gentle vacuum, molding the cornea to the engineered interior shape of the contact lens.

When hard contacts were initially developed, they were meant to be worn during the day. It took until 1994 to have the FDA grant approval for the first daily wear lens designed for orthokeratology, and another eight years before they granted approval for overnight wear. I gave the first-ever lecture on overnight wear lenses back in the 1970s. We had found that by using overnight lenses, there was no adaptation period. It allowed us to fit more patients, and they were able to sleep right through any discomfort they might have felt and still reap the benefits of orthokeratology.

The delay in getting FDA approval, I believe, was partially due to the eye-care community's traditional mindset against altering the shape of the cornea. "Optometrists, a famously conservative group whose bread and butter was fixing simple vision problems with traditional glasses or contacts, were leery of reshaping the eye. Ophthalmologists—surgery-minded medical school graduates—only wanted new and better invasive procedures… orthokeratology was derided as black magic" (*Los Angeles Magazine*, January 2004). Most eye doctors didn't seem to have an issue with cutting into the eye or burning away corneal tissue with lasers to permanently change the shape of the cornea. However, there was a huge reluctance to accept the process of non-invasively reshaping the cornea through the use of rigid contacts, which is something I still can't understand. There is no harm or downside to orthokeratology. It is almost impossible not to be successful.

Even today, surgery seems to be the only game in town. LASIK became popular because laser manufacturers contributed millions to advertising, so within six months, everyone knew about it. Most doctors still stick with traditional methods as it is much easier to fit patients with spectacles or soft contacts versus rigid contacts. Not only are soft contacts admittedly more comfortable, but some doctors fear the loss of recurring income by having their patients switch to rigid lenses. What they don't realize is that patients can go anywhere for glasses or soft contacts as long as they have a valid prescription. They can even order them online.

Some doctors claim that Ortho-K lenses are too expensive. However, when compared to the lifelong expense of monthly soft contacts, or the cost of treatment for eventual eye diseases or corrective surgery, Ortho-K is much more affordable, especially when you take into account the improvement to overall eye health. Regardless, the patients should be the ones to decide what is important to them. They should have the freedom to not have to depend on devices such as spectacles. Doctors should tell their patients about all of their options, even if a specific option isn't something that doctor specializes in. It is more important to help patients change who they were, liberating them from the inconvenience of corrective lenses.

Because Dr. May and I were practitioners, and not stuck in a lab, we got to see the results of our research firsthand. It has been extremely rewarding work. However, despite our successes and the clear benefits of Ortho-K, there still isn't a high percentage of doctors trained to fit patients with these custom lenses. Out of the forty thousand or so optometrists in the United States, only about five hundred fit patients with Ortho-K regularly.

Orthokeratology is advanced medical technology designed to help myopic patients, especially children, with their eyesight. It is not a one-size-fits-all procedure. It takes skill and experience. It takes a special practitioner to want to do it, the kind of person willing to go into new areas and keep learning, one who is dedicated to making the lives of patients better. It doesn't require the same level of skill to fit patients with traditional soft contacts. Since Ortho-K lenses are custom designed for each patient, special equipment and knowledge is needed to take measurements, to know whether the end product is what was ordered. While it is my sincere wish for more eye doctors to become trained in orthokeratology, I feel it is better to have fewer doing a good job than lots doing a mediocre job.

Orthokeratology is clearly a valuable option in treating myopia. It has the ability to slow the progression of myopia, provide perfect or near-perfect vision, and decrease the risk of eye diseases all while having virtually no side effects. Unlike other corrective procedures, the impact of Ortho-K lenses is completely reversible. If you decide you are unhappy with the results or that you no longer want to wear the lenses, you can simply stop. Within a couple of days, your vision will return to where it was prior to beginning the use of Ortho-K lenses. For example, if you wear Ortho-K lenses for ten years and then decide to stop for whatever reason, you will have preserved the health of your cornea and subsequently, your retina for that period of time. Even if your myopia begins to progress again once you stop wearing the Ortho-K lenses, you will have decreased your risk of eye diseases and retinal detachment by putting off the progression of the myopia.

Yet, even with all of these benefits, orthokeratology is still not mainstream. Why? I believe this is due to an overall lack of knowledge regarding myopia. My goal in contributing to this book is to help educate the public regarding their options. I firmly believe that orthokeratology is the solution to the growing epidemic of myopia in our country.

Part of our country's lack of knowledge stems from the media. The general public hears the news as opposed to the research. Several years ago, a number of children in China got severe eye infections that resulted in vision loss while using CRT (Corneal Reshaping Therapy) lenses. This story made headlines. However, follow-up research proved that the lenses were fine and it was the lack of proper education that led to this incident. The children were not instructed to properly clean their lenses, which led to the infections. Unlike the initial coverage of the incident, the follow-up research didn't make the news and those in opposition of Ortho-K continue to cite these news stories. While the fact remains that Ortho-K lenses do carry the risk of eye infections, the risk is no greater than with any other overnight lens and it can be greatly reduced by following proper care procedures.

The effectiveness of Ortho-K lenses has gone well beyond theoretical. Multiple studies have been conducted to support the benefits and effectiveness of these lenses. Although there are other options for controlling myopia, orthokeratology has been found to be highly effective as the following studies prove.

Longitudinal Orthokeratology Research in Children (LORIC)

The Longitudinal Orthokeratology Research in Children (LORIC) study, conducted by Cho and coworkers, worked with children in Hong Kong. This study compared a group of children using orthokeratology lenses and an age- and sex-matched group of children wearing glasses over the course of two years. After the two years, they found the group using orthokeratology lenses had significantly less progression in their axial elongation and their vitreous chamber depth than the group wearing glasses. Essentially, the children in glasses experienced a worsening in their myopia while the children in the orthokeratology lenses did not.

This research study supports the assertion that Ortho-K can effectively stop the progression of myopia while corrective lenses do not. The strain created by wearing daily corrective lenses impacts the elongation of the eye, which in turn increases the severity of the myopia. It is a vicious cycle because when vision decreases, stronger prescriptions are provided, which further worsens the patient's vision.

The Children's Overnight Orthokeratology Investigation (COOKI)

The Children's Overnight Orthokeratology Investigation (COOKI) was a six-month study into the effectiveness and safety of wearing overnight lenses. They found no serious negative events throughout the course of the study. The study came in the wake of an incident in China where several children developed severe eye infections while wearing Ortho-K lenses. This incident resulted in many believing the lenses were not safe. This study was also particularly important for the eventual mainstream use and acceptance of orthokeratology due to the fact it is being used primarily on children. There is always a certain level of weariness that needs to be addressed when a process or procedure is new.

There are some within the eye-health community who still assert that Ortho-K lenses are not safe, and they cite the case in China to back their claims. However, it was determined that the children in China impacted by that situation were not given proper cleaning and use instructions, which resulted in them cleaning their lenses with tap water. This is what led to the dramatic increase in eye infections at that time. Tap water, regardless of where it comes from, has minerals and often bacteria in it which can attach to the lens and be transferred to the eye.

Corneal Reshaping and Yearly Observation of Nearsightedness (CRAYON)

Following the COOKI study was the Corneal Reshaping and Yearly Observation of Nearsightedness (CRAYON) study. CRAYON compared two groups of age- and sex-matched children. One group wore orthokeratology lenses, and the control group wore soft contact lenses. At the end of the study, the orthokeratology group was found to have less axial length elongation and less of an increase in vitreous chamber depth. Similar to the LORIC study, the CRAYON study showed that the progression of myopia was significantly less with the use of Ortho-K. While these studies are very similar, they are equally important. It is through repeated research and consistent results that orthokeratology gains mainstream acceptance within the eye-care field.

Retardation of Myopia in Orthokeratology (ROMIO)

Retardation of myopia in Orthokeratology (ROMIO) was a two-year randomized clinical trial that focused solely on evaluating the effectiveness of Ortho-K lenses for controlling myopia. This study included 102 children between the ages of six and ten, who had myopia between -0.50 and -4.0D. The participants were randomly assigned to either wear Ortho-K lenses or glasses for a two-year period. The results of this study showed that the children wearing the Ortho-K lenses experienced a slower increase in axial elongation by 43 percent, compared to the group of children wearing glasses. Studies examining the effectiveness of Ortho-K lenses in slowing the progression of myopia have consistently demonstrated their effectiveness.

Stabilizing Myopia by Accelerated Reshaping Technique (SMART)

The Stabilizing Myopia by Accelerated Reshaping Technique (SMART) was a large multi-year study that compared reverse geometry overnight lenses with soft contacts worn during the day. The results of this study were promising and supported the findings of the other studies. This study, however, was conducted with adult participants. While many of the studies have been conducted with children, Ortho-K is a viable option for adults as well. As long as your vision is within the parameters for Ortho-K, it doesn't matter how old you are. All myopia patients can benefit from myopia-control measures.

Ortho-K Lenses and Vision-Related Quality-of-Life Measures

Another study conducted in Spain focused on the possible connection between myopia control with Ortho-K lenses and vision-related quality-of-life measures. To do this, researchers used participants ranging from six to twelve years old with myopia ranging from -0.75D to -4.00D. Each participant answered a pediatric refractive error profile questionnaire that explored the children's perceptions of overall vision, near vision, far distance vision, symptoms, appearance, satisfaction, activities, academic performance, handling, and peer perception. These questionnaires were completed at twelve- and twenty-four-month intervals. The children wearing the Ortho-K lenses reported a significantly higher perceptions in areas of overall vision, far distance vision, symptoms, appearance, satisfaction, activities, academic performance, and peer perception. These results demonstrate a clear improvement in vision-related quality-of-life measures for children with Ortho-K lenses.

The study on vision-related quality-of-life measures is particularly important because it demonstrates the greater impact poor eyesight has on children, as well as the intrinsic value of Ortho-K lenses. Later in this book, we will discuss in detail the impact poor eyesight can have on self-esteem and self-image amongst teenagers. This is a significant issue that needs to be considered in addition to the medical/visual benefits of Ortho-K lenses.

Each of these studies examined the effectiveness of orthokeratology as a means of slowing the progression of myopia. In addition, with proper care, orthokeratology lenses have been found to be safe and there are no short- or long-term negative complications associated with the use of these lenses.

Based on the research supporting the safety and effectiveness of Ortho-K lenses, it should be considered as a viable option for all those impacted by myopia. Orthokeratology accounts for more than 80 percent of my practice and I have helped several thousand patients see more clearly with orthokeratology over the course of my career. I've kept corneas in that position for forty years now. I take people who can't get out of bed in the morning without their glasses, and I get them down to a 20/40 or a 20/50. Their vision may not be perfect but at least they have the freedom and flexibility to know that if they don't wear anything, they can still function.

I may not get every patient's eyesight to where they want it, but we can improve their lives. People have asked me if I cured the myopia. I don't know, but I've kept my patients from needing to wear glasses. I can't make everybody perfect, but I can make everybody better, especially children. Orthokeratology is one of the only methods of myopia control that is safe for children. And with the rest of their lives ahead of them, controlling their myopia now will preserve their vision in the future.

CHAPTER TEN

Who Benefits From Ortho-K?

It has already been established that long-term myopia is a dangerous condition due to the increased risk of eye diseases and retinal detachment. However, there are a wide range of other reasons patients may benefit from Ortho-K lenses. With the variety of eye-health conditions in this country, it is important to understand who can benefit from Ortho-K. In truth, anyone dealing with nearsightedness can gain clearer vision and stop the progression of myopia with this method of control. However, to provide a clearer picture, we will discuss the different types of patients and lifestyles most likely to benefit from Ortho-K lenses.

Myopia is the only prerequisite when determining if a patient qualifies for orthokeratology. As doctors, we work with all sorts of patients, who have any number of reasons for not wanting to rely on glasses or contacts any more. While there are some cases where patients are not helped by Ortho-K, this is typically due to the extreme condition of their eyes, such as advanced eye diseases or permanent vision loss. Even patients with severe myopia can benefit from Ortho-K. Their vision may not become perfect, but they can gain clearer sight without the risks and side effects of more invasive methods.

With myopia quickly becoming an epidemic in this country, this book focuses mainly on the benefits of orthokeratology for children. However, adults can certainly benefit from this technology as well.

Active kids: Having to dealing with glasses while participating in any kind of sport or vigorous activity can be frustrating, and is even more so for children. Kids are constantly on the go and don't want to be burdened with glasses continually slipping, sliding, flopping, and falling off. Every time your children jump, their glasses go flying out of place or off their faces completely. Jumping rope, swinging, doing somersaults, playing sports, running; these are just some of the activities that can cause children to lose or break their glasses.

Sweating from running around and playing also makes it even harder for children to keep their glasses in place. Not only does the extra moisture cause their glasses to fog up, reducing their vision, but they are constantly having to push their glasses up or taking them off to do things, which increases the chances of lost or broken glasses.

Active kids are much more likely to break their glasses than kids who spend most of their time indoors. However, spending time outside is one of the best ways of controlling the progression of myopia. Fear of breaking or losing their glasses shouldn't keep kids from playing and being active outside.

Active kids who participate in team sports typically need to wear athletic goggles during most sporting events. Goggles with a high prescription stand out even more than regular glasses, which can increase the child's chances of being bullied. Ortho-K lenses give active kids the freedom to play as much as they want, without any of the worries associated with glasses or contacts.

Studious kids: Like all kids with glasses, studious kids don't want their eyes to continually get worse. They don't want the increased risk of blindness later in life or to feel different or get bullied at school. Studious children don't want to have to constantly take their glasses on and off when they read, do work, or sit at a computer, increasing the likelihood of losing or breaking their glasses.

Research has shown that children with high achievement in school are more likely to develop myopia, and are therefore, at greater risk of eye diseases and blindness later in life. Clearly, stopping kids from reading and studying is not an option. Controlling their myopia with the use of Ortho-K lenses can stop the progression and preserve their overall eye health.

Now that I wear Ortho-K lenses, I have better eyesight, which helps me in school.
– Iris C.

Active adults: Similar to active children, active adults often feel burdened by their glasses, taking them on and off constantly to readjust, clean them, wipe the sweat from their brow, and so on. No one wants to be out working in their yard, playing a sport, building a fire, bird-watching, or exercising, and constantly having to adjust their glasses or push them up.

Since Ortho-K lenses reshape your cornea while you sleep, you wake up each morning with clearer vision. Whatever the day might throw at you, you won't have to worry about adjusting your glasses or the possibility of eye irritation due to soft contacts.

Teens: It is important to understand that many of the personal, self-image, and self-esteem ramifications of wearing glasses and having bad eyesight really hit hardest during the teen years. Multiple studies have been conducted examining the connection between poor vision and self-esteem. These studies have shown the negative impact poor vision can have on a teenager, regardless of the recent increase in the social acceptance of glasses.

In addition to self-image and self-esteem issues, teenagers who are very active, athletic, or studious will experience all the additional challenges associated with wearing glasses. Many young people also learn to drive during their teenage years. Having crisp, clear, and unencumbered vision is essential while driving, especially for new drivers who are already at an increased risk of danger when behind the wheel. Ortho-K lenses reduce the need for glasses, allowing teenagers to focus on other aspects of their lives.

> *Ortho-K lenses have helped me with my eyesight and all the other challenges that come with competing in a sport that requires excellent vision in some difficult conditions. With their help, I was able to become the state Skeet champion. – Kyle J.*

Workers: There is an endless list of jobs and positions that are made more difficult or even impossible when the person has to rely on glasses or contacts. For example, one of my earliest patients was a pilot who wanted to avoid relying on contacts. He knew that if one of his contacts slipped out during a flight, he would be left unable to see clearly and could potentially endanger the entire plane. I also worked with a man who wanted to be a firefighter but couldn't pass the eye exam.

Jobs that require the use of dust or ventilation masks are also more difficult when the wearer must depend on glasses. Many jobs require safety goggles, which means those with glasses either need to get goggles that are big enough to fit over their spectacles or get prescription safety glasses. Airline pilots, police officers, paramedics, doctors, surgeons—these are all positions that rely on clear vision. If their glasses fall off or their contacts slip out of place, negatively impacting their vision at the wrong time, lives could be in danger. Not only do Ortho-K lenses allow patients to pursue careers otherwise off-limits to them, but they give those patients the ability to perform their jobs safely and accurately.

> *I was very skeptical about whether Ortho-K would work for me. I thought that sleeping with hard lenses would be very uncomfortable, and I didn't think they would be able to match the clarity I had with the soft lenses. With Ortho-K, however, I don't have a problem sleeping with the lenses in, and I am seeing better than 20/20. In law enforcement, I rely on my vision a great deal. Ortho-K has exceeded my expectations, and I don't have to wear contact lenses during my shift. – Manny*

Busy mothers: Mothers, especially new mothers, are constantly on the go and regularly faced with unexpected and often messy situations. Being able to go through the day and handle everything that happens without having to constantly clean and adjust their glasses means they have one less thing to deal with. Mothers with young children also have to deal with their little ones constantly grabbing their glasses right off their faces, often resulting in the glasses getting damaged.

Mothers typically don't enjoy a regular sleep schedule, which makes contacts difficult to deal with as well. Those who do rely on contacts likely find themselves sleeping with their contacts in more and more often, which isn't advised unless the contacts are specifically designed to do so. Many mothers end up splitting their time between wearing glasses and contacts for convenience. Ortho-K alleviates all these issues by reducing their reliance on corrective lenses entirely during the day.

Those who aren't candidates for corrective surgery: Orthokeratology provides a safe alternative to laser eye surgery. While both methods eliminate the need for glasses or contacts, Ortho-K doesn't have any of the risks associated with laser eye surgery. It is successful in most patients, and is effective long-term. As long as you continue wearing the overnight lenses, you will continue enjoying the daytime benefits of better vision.

Only a specific and select group of people are good candidates for laser eye surgery. However, almost anyone with myopia is a candidate for Ortho-K. While Ortho-K is not successful in 100 percent of patients, the success rate is very high, and for those who do not find success, there are other options for myopia control that may work.

Who Benefits From Ortho-K?

Those afraid of corrective surgery: Laser eye surgery carries some serious risks. For those who end up with unsuccessful laser eye surgery, the impact is long-term. There are multiple potential complications, including ongoing dryness and irritation. In some cases, the surgery can result in permanent deterioration of vision. While many laser eye surgery patients benefit greatly and experience no complications, the risks are real and need to be considered.

Another factor to consider in regard to laser eye surgery is that surgery does not stop the progression of myopia. While it may correct your vision currently, myopia can still reoccur and progress. You may need to go back to corrective lenses or have follow-up surgery in the future. Ortho-K, on the other hand, can give most myopic patients clearer vision without the risks associated with laser eye surgery. New research also shows that Ortho-K is effective in controlling the progression of myopia in patients who have already had LASIK but their eyes are getting worse.

> *I'm glad I decided to try Ortho-K! More than ten years ago, I had LASIK surgery to correct my myopia. After the second year, the myopia started to come back and with my first pregnancy it got worse. I was told I could have the surgery done again, but I did not trust it would work since my vision was not stable. Then I saw an interview on TV about Ortho-K and decided to give it a try. Although the doctor explained that the lenses were not guaranteed to work for eye surgery patients, I went for it. I have been wearing them for the last four years and I love them! I put them on when going to sleep and take them off when waking up, and I see perfectly fine during the whole day. Even better, my prescription has not changed since I started wearing the lenses. – Ana R.*

Professionals, sales professionals, and executives: Teenagers aren't the only ones impacted by negative self-image or self-esteem issues. For individuals working in professional or executive positions, their jobs require them to constantly interact with others and provide a level of authority and self-confidence. Wearing glasses can impact the way you see yourself and how you are viewed by others. You may not like the way you look in glasses, or feel they don't project the image you want to portray.

Ortho-K lenses eliminate these concerns. Since the lenses are worn at night, they don't impact your daily interactions.

Athletes: Athletes who wear glasses typically have to rely on athletic goggles when participating in sports. Although athletic goggles work, they can be very uncomfortable, especially when an athlete is hot and sweating. Wearing contacts while playing sports can cause problems as well, particularly when sweat gets in an athlete's eyes and causes the contacts to get blurry or results in irritation. Additionally, if the contacts slip, fall out, or get blurry during a vital part of a game or competition, it can negatively impact the athlete's performance.

Laser eye surgery is an option, but if it is unsuccessful, it could mean the end of an athlete's career. Ortho-K lenses are safe, effective, and carry almost none of the side-effects inherent with laser eye surgery. The results are also completely reversible should the patient decide to stop wearing the lenses in the future.

> *I began using Ortho-K lenses as an athlete in high school. They gave me perfect vision without the disadvantages of glasses or daytime contacts. I could finally hit a curveball again. Ortho-K lenses have since slowed the development of my astigmatism and allowed me to appreciate everything from the intricate patterns or a snowflake to the ornate carvings of Ankor Wat. It's been over ten years, and I still use Ortho-K lenses regularly. – Jared K.*

Those who prefer natural remedies: Although laser eye surgery has become relatively common, there are a lot of people who prefer not to undergo elective surgeries. All surgeries carry risks, and the easiest way to avoid those risks is to avoid having surgery altogether. Additionally, some of the potential negative complications of laser eye surgery can only be corrected with additional surgeries.

Controlling the progression of myopia with Ortho-K lenses will dramatically decrease or even eliminate the potential for future eye surgeries related to the diseases and conditions that can develop, such as cataracts, retinal detachment, and glaucoma. These conditions, if detected early enough, can only be treated through surgery. Ortho-K is the clear choice for patients with myopia who want to avoid not only elective eye surgery, but potentially necessary eye surgery later in life.

Those afraid of needles: For people who are afraid of needles, the thought of any kind of surgery is terrifying, with laser eye surgery even more so. The thought of being wide awake while a surgeon cuts into their eye is incredibly overwhelming. However, that doesn't mean they are destined to wear corrective lenses the rest of their lives.

Ortho-K offers a safe, painless, and needle-free alternative to laser eye surgery. Since the use of Ortho-K lenses may also slow or stop the progression of myopia, it can potentially eliminate the need for necessary eye surgery in the future. Another potential advantage for Ortho-K is that it may keep your child's vision at a lower prescription which could allow them to opt for LASIK in the future if they so choose. The higher the prescription, the less likely they will be a good candidate for LASIK.

Those who dislike glasses or contacts: There are dozens of reasons someone may hate wearing glasses or contacts. In addition to the discomfort and inconvenience associated with glasses mentioned earlier, another reason to consider is cost. As your prescription increases, the more expensive it becomes to make your glasses thinner and lighter. However, regardless of the reason, Ortho-K can alleviate these concerns by providing clear vision without the need for daytime corrective lenses. While Ortho-K does require the patient to wear overnight lenses, the fact that they are worn only at night eliminates many of the concerns patients have with wearing traditional corrective lenses.

Corrected vision, without the need for sweaty, pinching, awkward glasses OR itchy, dry contacts! I would recommend Ortho-K lenses to everyone, definitely! – Janine G.

Those prone to redness, dryness, irritation, and blurriness from daytime contacts: I have had many patients over the years who regularly have to switch between their glasses and contacts. They either can't wear their contacts all day due to the irritation they cause, or they can wear their contacts for a few days but then need to switch to their glasses to give their eyes a break.

Soft contacts can cause redness, dryness, irritation, and blurriness in some patients, making it uncomfortable for them to wear their contacts for extended periods of time. These symptoms can become so severe that patients are forced to take their contacts out at random times. However, orthokeratology allows patients to go without glasses or contacts during the day. Wearing Ortho-K lenses while you sleep decreases and often eliminates the potential for these symptoms.

Those tired of the complications associated with contacts: Soft contacts essentially float on the surface of your eye. This allows them to easily move with your eye as you look around. However, contacts can sometimes slip out of place or fall out completely. People who rely on daytime contacts have to carry around contact solution, a contact case, and their glasses—just in case such an occurrence happens.

Women who wear eye makeup cannot safely and hygienically put their contacts back in during the day without first washing away their eye makeup. Any dirt from their hands can be transferred to the contact lens when they try to put it back in their eye. They need to be near a clean bathroom with backup supplies, so they can clean their hands and the contact before putting it back in. Finding the right facilities and making sure you have the necessary supplies on hand is not only frustrating but inconvenient. Most women end up just doing the best they can with the situation they are in.

As mentioned earlier, depending on when and where your contacts slip or fall out, it can put you or others in danger. This isn't just a risk for airline pilots, doctors, or police officers. Losing a contact while driving, riding a bike, lifting or moving something heavy, or playing sports can cause anyone to get injured or possibly injure someone else. Orthokeratology is ideal for patients who are tired of dealing with daytime contacts by giving them the freedom of clear vision without the reliance on corrective lenses.

> *It's a MIRACLE! In my wildest dreams, I never envisioned (see that pun) that I would be able to wake up and see clearly without my contact lenses or my glasses ALL day and evening long. My vision is even better now than when I was wearing my contact lenses. I have extremely tender eyeballs and found even my soft contact lenses to be irritating quite often. I was always ready to remove them by the end of the day. It is so wonderful to be able to wake up, pop out my Ortho-K lenses, hop in the shower, and see clearly. As a person not able to see the large E on the vision chart clearly, it is amazing to be able to see so well in all situations. I just put them back in at bedtime, close my eyes, and wake up still maintaining my good vision. I have told several friends and colleagues about this amazing therapy and am happy to report that they are considering it, as they, like myself, are still not ready to contemplate laser vision surgery. – Maggie*

Self-conscious individuals: The available choices of eyeglass frames have grown exponentially in recent years. Many people have even started to see glasses as an accessory, wearing different pairs depending on their moods or outfits. However, not everyone sees the use of correctives lenses as fashionable.

No matter how fancy the glasses are, some people simply don't like the way they look in glasses. They don't like how their face is partially hidden or how glasses hide their eye makeup. They don't like the shadows the frames can cast on their face. There are plenty of reasons someone may not like the way they look in glasses. However, regardless of the reason, orthokeratology allows for clear vision without the need to wear glasses.

Swimmers: Swimming has always been a challenge for people who wear corrective lenses. You can't swim with your glasses on because they can hurt your face, fall off, and can easily get lost in the water. When wet, they are also hard to see through, due to water droplets and fogging. Taking them off before going in the pool leaves you with poor vision. You can't fully enjoy your surroundings, interact with others, keep track of your kids, or spot potential dangers.

Likewise, contacts can't be worn in water either. The chlorine in swimming pools can negatively impact the lenses, causing blurriness, itching, redness, and irritation. However, it isn't only the chlorine that poses a problem. The water from lakes, rivers, the ocean, and even your tap can carry impurities that can lead to eye infection. Normally, your tears help wash away these impurities, but wearing soft contacts can inhibit the flow of tears and trap those impurities in your eye.

Since Ortho-K lenses eliminate the need for glasses or contacts during the day, swimming and other water activities become enjoyable again. There is no longer a need to worry about blurry vision or eye infections when spending the day at the pool or beach.

> *Within the first week, I could see 20/20. Being able to get in the car and drive without contacts or glasses is unbelievable. I've worn glasses since I was fourteen and contacts since I was seventeen, and this is amazing. I was in the pool yesterday and could look out and see the pine cones with such clarity. I swam underwater and did not hit the wall. – Eillen*

Book lovers: The increased prevalence of myopia has been connected to the recent increased reliance on near work. This not only includes the use of electronic devices and computers, but reading as well. A study conducted in Alaska focused on elderly individuals and their grandchildren. The primary difference between the two groups was that the elderly participants were all illiterate while the younger participants could read. The results showed that the younger group had a prevalence of myopia comparable to other parts of the country, yet the elderly group had a prevalence in the single digits.

With the use of Ortho-K lenses, myopic patients can stabilize their vision and continue to enjoy near work activities like reading without having to worry about damaging their vision. Since Ortho-K may also decrease the risk of future eye diseases and other conditions, it allows patients the freedom to pursue their passions as they age.

People with allergies: Seasonal allergy sufferers often get itchy, dry and irritated eyes for several weeks at a time. They may find themselves rubbing their eyes more often, and many need to use eye drops to alleviate their symptoms. Many people who normally wear contacts have to switch to their glasses during allergy season to help control the irritation and be able to use allergy drops as most eye drops can't be used with contacts.

Since Ortho-K lenses reduce the need for both glasses and contacts, switching between them during allergy season is no longer necessary.

People who use magnifying lenses or microscopes for work or recreation: It doesn't matter if you are a doctor, scientist, astronomer, or an avid bird watcher, wearing glasses makes it very difficult to properly see through any kind of magnifying lens. Magnifying lenses like microscopes, telescopes, and binoculars work best when you can look through them with your naked eye. The same applies to traditional cameras.

Using magnifying lenses is actually what first attracted me to learning about orthokeratology. I found it frustrating to have to constantly remove and adjust my glasses to see through the microscope when conducting eye examinations on my patients. Ortho-K lenses have allowed many of my patients to use magnifying lenses either for work or recreation without being encumbered by glasses.

Parents and Guardians: Even if the parents and guardians of myopic children are not myopic themselves, they can still benefit from Ortho-K lenses. By providing Ortho-K lenses for their children, parents benefit by helping preserve their child's eye health and allowing them freedom from glasses and contacts.

Many believe that myopia control is merely a way to avoid wearing glasses. While there are clear benefits to not having to wear glasses or contacts, it is important to remember that the core benefit comes from decreasing the risks associated with myopia by controlling its progression. If told when their child was only six years old that the child could be blind by the time he or she reached fifty due to a retinal detachment, no doubt any parent would do whatever he or she could to prevent that from happening.

Every child diagnosed as myopic and prescribed corrective lenses is at a potentially increased risk for conditions like retinal detachment. Better education of parents is essential to controlling the epidemic of myopia that the world is currently facing. Knowing that you have the power to protect your children's vision as they age and even grow old is crucial.

With all these benefits of Ortho-K lenses, are there people who do not make good candidates? This is an important question to consider. While Ortho-K can help the majority of people with myopia, it won't work for everyone. For example, Ortho-K requires a healthy cornea. If your cornea has significant scars or other issues, it may not be strong enough for Ortho-K to work.

Properly cleaning and handling the lenses is vital in preventing severe eye infections. Therefore, people with poor hygiene or an inability to handle the lenses, such as extremely young or extremely old patients, are not good candidates. Also, those who suffer from frequent and severe dry eye, inflammation, infections, or other eye problems may not be good candidates for Ortho-K.

Despite these limitations, anyone with myopia should consult with their doctor about improving their vision with Ortho-K. Even if you think you may not be a good candidate, an optometrist trained in orthokeratology can examine your eyes and discuss your options with you.

There is certainly something very freeing about being able to see clearly and naturally without having to worry about glasses or contacts. Yet, having that freedom from corrective lenses is one many adults and children don't get to enjoy. Now, with orthokeratology, there is an alternative in myopia control.

CHAPTER ELEVEN

The Benefits of Ortho-K for Children

The health benefits of orthokeratology and myopia control have been clearly established through research for both children and adults. However, the benefits are especially important for children. One in every four children has an undetected vision problem. Starting the use of Ortho-K lenses as soon as a child is diagnosed as myopic provides the best immediate and long-term benefits. The child's current vision will be corrected, and his or her threat of future vision loss will be greatly diminished.

Aside from the medical benefits, there are also social and emotional benefits of Ortho-K for children. Extensive research has been conducted to demonstrate the potential impact poor vision and the use of corrective lenses can have on a child's self-image, self-esteem, confidence, perceived ability, and educational performance. There have also been multiple studies conducted on how children tend to stereotype other children who wear glasses. While the social acceptance of glasses has increased greatly over recent decades, studies have shown that children with glasses are more likely to be bullied than those without. Poor vision and a reliance on glasses can also impact a child's ability to learn in many ways. It can lead to the misdiagnosis of learning disabilities, and can also exacerbate the impact of learning disabilities in children, making education more frustrating. Vision and the ability to learn are connected in a multitude of ways. Through research, it has been discovered that the negative impact of myopia extends far beyond the physical effects it has on the eyes.

Vision-Related Issues in Young Children

Poor vision can be difficult to detect in children who are nonverbal or too young to adequately communicate how they feel and what they are experiencing.

The symptoms of poor vision in very young children are also often overlooked by pediatricians. The doctors are usually more interested in how the children behave while playing or interacting with others.

Signs of poor vision in very young children:
- Bringing objects very close to the eyes
- Holding the head in a strange position when trying to focus on something
- Limited eye contact (meaning the child does not hold another person's gaze for very long)
- Constantly rubbing the eyes
- Reaching for something and missing it
- Failing to look directly at the object the child is trying to see

When children display any of these signs of poor vision, two things are happening. First, the child is not getting the opportunity to really enjoy everything that is going on around him or her. They are limited by what they can see and what they can interact with closely. In the early years, children learn a great deal simply by observing and interacting with the world around them. Poor vision can negatively impact the way your child learns at this young age.

Second, the child is learning to compensate for his or her diminished vision, which can create bad habits and may delay the detection of poor vision. For example, a child may bring things closer to his or her face in order to see it or squint at distant objects, both common adaptations. Children adapt without understanding why they need to do these things. If they realized they were doing these things to accommodate for their poor vision, and that how they see is not optimal, they could simply tell a parent. However, they are too young to comprehend that and, without knowing what clear vision is like, they don't realize they have a problem.

Having poor vision from a young age impacts the way children behave, learn, and interact with others. It can lead to an inadequate understanding of nonverbal communication, which can lead to social awkwardness and shyness causing them to feel they don't fit in. A lot of young patients are severely introverted. They tend to be very quiet and shy, and they stay close to their parents throughout their exams. They may hide their faces when asked a direct question. By the time we get their vision corrected, they are more talkative, outgoing, and interactive with me throughout the appointment. I've seen this change in young patients over and over again.

These changes in personality are a result of their improved vision. They are able to gain confidence in social settings because they can finally take in everything going on around them. They no longer miss nonverbal cues and can participate more fully with the world around them. They learn more, and that increased knowledge fuels their newfound confidence. I am always delighted to work with young children who get to experience clear vision, possibly for the first time.

Vision-Related School Issues

Poor vision in children has been linked to a number of learning and behavioral problems. The first step to understanding if a particular issue is vision related is to identify whether your school-age child does indeed have poor vision. It is often hard to detect because the symptoms can overlap with other learning and behavioral problems. Until something is done to correct their vision, children with poor eyesight do not know the difference, so it is not something they are typically able to articulate.

Poor vision has been associated with the following issues in school:
- Short attention span
- Hyperactivity
- Talking
- Disrupting class
- Refusal to read or do class work
- Not following directions
- Not working well with others
- Not able to play or study quietly
- Getting angry easily
- Lacking motivation
- Displaying poor organizational skills
- Regularly forgetting or losing homework

As I mentioned, these behaviors can be attributed to any number of learning, behavioral, or social problems, which is why it is not always clear when a child is suffering from poor vision. Most schools do not start checking children's vision until they are in the second grade, sometimes even older. Additionally, school-based vision testing is generally very limited. Unless a child has severe myopia, it can often still go undetected. While it may seem like not all of these behavioral issues would be linked to poor vision, multiple studies have demonstrated a connection.

In addition to behavioral problems, poor vision can also cause:
- Headaches
- Eyestrain
- Fatigue
- Burning eyes
- Itching and watery eyes
- Poor hand-eye coordination
- Poor memory and concentration

Dealing with the complications of poor vision can be extremely frustrating for children. As that frustration builds, it can lead to anger, aggression, poor self-esteem, and low self-confidence. These feelings can lead to behavioral and discipline issues at school, which will only fuel the frustration more.

Social and Emotional Impact of Glasses on Children

The problems associated with poor vision in children are not limited to those with undetected vision problems. While wearing glasses can certainly correct poor vision and help the child overcome related learning issues, the glasses themselves can cause a host of other problems. Being able to see clearly may also decrease the frustration, anger, and behavioral problems that children often demonstrate; however, wearing glasses comes with its own frustrations.

According to a paper published in the *European Jounral of Developmental Psychology*, children often link glasses with negative traits, which can lead to bullying and stereotyping as mentioned earlier. These negative traits aren't limited to those of their peers, but how children view themselves as well. This study found that a vast majority of children are afraid of having to wear glasses because of how they will look and how other children will treat them.

Despite the increased acceptance of glasses in recent years, they can still create a social division. Unfortunately, the differences in appearance between those who wear glasses and those who don't often lead to categorizing. Even if their peers are accepting, children may choose to separate themselves, feeling they are different because they wear glasses.

Another study focused on children between the ages of five and nine years old. Each participant looked at pictures of other children, some wearing glasses and some not. The pictures of children wearing glasses were typically labeled as *worse looking*, while the pictures of the children without glasses were labeled as *prettier*. These results show that children associate glasses with a lack of attractiveness. Despite the fact this study focused on relatively young children, there was still a clear division. Wearing glasses can impact a child's perceived attractiveness.

In another study, the children looked at pictures of other children wearing glasses and were asked whether they thought the child in the picture looked cute, friendly, well-behaved, or smart. Overall, the feedback from the participants was negative. The only exception was that the female participants were more likely to say the children with glasses looked friendlier.

A 2008 study found that children between the ages of six and ten tended to stereotype children in glasses as being smarter. While some may argue that being classified as smarter is not a negative attribute, anytime children get stereotyped, there are negative consequences. The smart stereotype can also lead to negative self-perception in children with a learning disability. They may feel they are expected to perform better academically than they actually do.

Numerous studies have also been done on the self-perception of children who wear glasses as opposed to children who don't. One study focused on children between the ages of eight and twelve and found that children who went from wearing glasses to contacts perceived themselves as more attractive and athletically-skilled after switching to contacts.

The older children are, the more likely they will be to not wear their glasses. They are more likely to want contacts, or to fear being bullied. Refusing to wear their glasses, particularly during school, can lead to decreased academic performance, as well as the concerns associated with undiagnosed poor vision mentioned earlier.

Adolescence can be a hard time for many kids. Children want to be accepted by their peers, which includes fitting in. They don't want to be labeled as different. The younger the child is when they are diagnosed with myopia, the greater the likelihood that there won't be many other children in their class who wear glasses. For some children, it may be novel at first. They may enjoy the idea of wearing glasses or standing out among their peers, but research shows the majority of children just feel singled out.

Learning Disabilities and Vision

It is important to understand the difference between learning disabilities and learning-related vision problems. According to the U.S. Individuals with Disabilities Education Act (IDEA), a learning disability is ...*a disorder in one or more of the basic psychological processes involved in understanding or in using language, spoken or written, that may manifest itself in an imperfect ability to listen, think, speak, read, write, spell, or do mathematical calculations, including conditions such as perceptual disabilities, brain injury, minimal brain dysfunction, dyslexia, and developmental aphasia.*

By this definition, a learning problem caused by poor vision is not considered a learning disability. That being said, a child may have a hard time learning and struggle academically due to a specific learning disability, a learning-related vision problem, or both. Helping your child is dependent on determining the root problem.

There are three types of learning-related vision problems: refractive problems, functional vision problems, and perceptual vision problems. Myopia is classified as a refractive problem since light that enters the eye does not bend (refract) correctly due to the elongation of the eyeball. Myopia directly impacts the child's ability to learn by making distant objects out of focus. Providing the child with corrective lenses will decrease or even eliminate the impact of myopia on their learning.

However, new concerns arise in the social and emotional issues children experience when wearing glasses. Additionally, the benefits of glasses are only present when the child is wearing them, so if your child resists wearing his or her glasses, breaks them, or regularly loses them, they can still end up dealing with their learning-related vision problem. This creates a cycle of learning, social, and emotional issues that frequently arises for children who have to wear glasses.

Another situation that can occur is the combination of a specific learning disability and a learning-related vision problem. For example, a child may be dyslexic and myopic at the same time. Dyslexia is a serious learning disability that makes it difficult for a child to read, write, and comprehend what they are reading. Although dyslexia is not curable, there are methods for teaching children how to cope with their dyslexia. Learning to read can be a difficult process for any child, and dyslexia only makes it more so. When dyslexia is combined with myopia, learning can become extremely frustrating.

Athletic Performance

Poor vision, as well as a dependence on corrective lenses, may also negatively impact children who play sports. Regardless of whether it is a simply game of kickball on the playground or an organized team sport, poor vision can lower a child's athletic performance by limiting his or her ability to see the surrounding environment. Poor vision impacts athletic ability in several ways. It:
- Makes it difficult for children to see across a field or playing area.
- Makes it difficult for children to focus on balls or other objects flying through the air.
- Can negatively impact a child's depth perception.
- Can make children hesitant and more afraid of getting injured.

Sports and other outdoor play are essential to every child's health and development. If a child struggles with a sport or is not very good at playing due to poor vision, he or she will be less inclined to play, causing the child to become more introverted. It may lead to embarrassment and a dislike for playing sports. By the time a child's vision is corrected, it may be too late to really embrace sports again.

Research has found that even with corrective lenses, poor vision can negatively impact a child's participation in sports and other outdoor games. Children who wear glasses are perceived as nonathletic. They are more likely to be chosen last for team sports, and may be discouraged to interact.

The increased fear of injury is also a concern for children who wear glasses. Since they may worry about breaking or losing their glasses while playing, they may be more likely to not wear their glasses, increasing their chances of falling or tripping. This fear can also decrease the child's willingness to take risks while playing sports, which negatively impacts their performance. As children get older, there is an expectation during athletic events that they should be completely focused on what they need to do to win. If young athletes are afraid of breaking their glasses, they will tend to be less aggressive.

While self-perception is shown to be higher in children who wear contacts versus glasses, wearing contacts can still impact their ability to play sports. Sweating, running, and participating in aggressive physical contact sports can cause an athlete to lose their contacts or have their contacts slip out of place.

Both instances can cause them to lose focus on what they are doing, potentially resulting in injury to themselves or others. Additionally, sweat can make contacts blurry and irritated.

Benefits of Ortho-K for Children

All of the social, emotional, and learning problems associated with myopia and the use of corrective lenses can be alleviated with orthokeratology. Ortho-K can provide children with perfect vision without the need for corrective lenses, allowing them to be able to see more clearly, learn more easily, and avoid the frustration of learning problems.

Here is what some teenaged patients had to say about their experiences with Ortho-K:

By my first night (or should I say morning), my vision had noticeably gotten better. It's been about four weeks now, and my vision is better than 20/20, which is normal vision. The contacts also helped with school and fun activities. They make things so much easier, because now in sports I can see what's going on without squinting. If I'd had regular contacts, I would not be able to open my eyes under water while swimming. Or something might get in my eye and bother me while trying to shoot the ball in basketball. But it not only helps in sports. After my vision was better, I was able to read the words on the overhead projectors and blackboards at school. I could then take better notes, and my grades got better! Before, I had NEVER been able to read the board. Everything is so much clearer and in so much more detail. It's amazing to see things I never saw before. – Amber

Orthokeratology has really transformed my life. After I started Ortho-K I had perfect vision in less than a week. I have perfect 20/20 vision in both eyes now, and I used to have 20/425 in the right eye and 20/375 in the left eye. The contact lenses are really easy to put in and even easier to take out and clean. It takes me about three minutes to put them in and about ten seconds to take them out and I am still improving. You don't even feel the lenses while you sleep. Orthokeratology has really improved my surfing ability. I can now actually see the waves and determine when it will break, and whether I should go for it. In golf, my game has definitely improved. My putting is better because it is easier to read the greens without glasses, and I can see the ball clearer after I hit it. My average golf tournament score used to be around 83 or 84 (about 11 or 12 over par). Ever since I started orthokeratology, I had my four best tournament scores, and my average tournament score since beginning Ortho-K is 79 (7 over par). In basketball, my shooting is superior to what it was, and my percentage has improved drastically. I even made fifty free throws in a row one day.

The most important thing that orthokeratology has given me is an increase in confidence and a positive personality. I hated wearing glasses so I only wore them while playing sports or in class, but outside of class everything was a blur. I could hardly see anything clearly, and I was always squinting, which made my eyes tired at the end of the day. During PE, I changed from being a poor football player to being one of the best in class just because I was able to see the ball. Also, while skiing, I had to wear glasses under my ski goggles so I could see, which was uncomfortable and bothersome, but now I just wear my goggles and feel great. In the end, orthokeratology has positively changed my life in so many ways and I would recommend it to anyone who has bad vision or doesn't like wearing glasses. I normally don't like to write, and when I do I don't write too much, but this long testimonial just goes to show how much I love orthokeratology and how it has positively affected me and changed my life. – Max

The freedom that comes with using Ortho-K lenses is a significant benefit for children of all ages, not just teens. Children who use Ortho-K are less likely to be bullied or stereotyped. They are more likely to have higher self-esteem as well as a higher perceived ability and attractiveness. In a perfect world, children would not stereotype or judge other children based on whether or not they wear glasses. Children would not determine their own ability or attractiveness based on their appearance. However, we are not living in a perfect world. By alleviating the need for corrective lenses, Ortho-K can eliminate a significant source of separation among children.

If your child has a learning disability in addition to myopia, the use Ortho-K lenses can eliminate the negative impact myopia has on his or her ability to learn. Ortho-K can make it easier for your child to adapt and provide him or her with one less factor to deal with, helping alleviate some of the stress you may feel as a parent.

In addition to these benefits, Ortho-K can also slow down or even stop the progression of your child's myopia, preserving his or her future vision by reducing the risk of retinal detachment and a variety of other ocular diseases.

What do you give your child when you gift them with clear vision through Ortho-K?

- Confidence
- Higher self-esteem
- Positive self-image
- Help in school
- Relief from constant frustration
- Better grades
- Reduced eye-health risks
- A better understanding of their eye health
- Better physical and athletic performance
- Better social interactions
- Reduced shyness

Benefits for Parents of Myopic Children

When one's child is struggling in school, when a child is withdrawn, not making friends easily, or being picked on, a parent wants to make everything better. While there are many things that may be out of your control, the negative impact of poor vision and corrective lenses is not one of them.

By improving your child's vision with Ortho-K, you can help him or her do better in school, feel more confident, and develop a positive self-image. However, the benefits don't end there. Correcting your child's vision now, will help him or her in a multitude of ways over the course of his or her entire life as the benefits of Ortho-K can extend well into your child's adult years. By teaching your child how to consistently and hygienically care for their lenses, you are also providing him or her with important lessons in responsibility. Your child can apply these skills to other areas of personal care, academics, and life.

If your child has been diagnosed as nearsighted, don't assume that glasses or soft contacts are the only option. Ask your eye doctor about orthokeratology. If your doctor doesn't offer Ortho-K, ask for a recommendation for another doctor in your area who does. A consultation is all you need to determine if your child is a candidate for Ortho-K. By exploring all of your options, you are setting your child on the right track for clear vision, good eye health, strong physical and academic performance, and self-confidence. Offering your child these advantages at a young age, when your child is developing both mentally and emotionally, will provide immeasurable benefits that will last a lifetime.

CHAPTER TWELVE

The Benefits of Ortho-K for Adults

While the benefits of Ortho-K are especially important for children, since managing their myopia now will preserve their eye health as they grow older, adults can certainly benefit as well. Often, eye doctors who specialize in Ortho-K promote it so much for children that it can leave parents feeling like the benefits don't apply to them. However, this couldn't be farther from the truth.

While it is true that Ortho-K cannot reverse the elongation that has already occurred in adult eyes, using the lenses may prevent further elongation and correct the current symptoms. Just as with children, adults can also experience perfect or near-perfect vision within just a few days of wearing Ortho-K lenses. This means no longer having to rely on glasses or contacts to drive, work, read, watch TV, or just get around your house.

Orthokeratology may significantly reduce your risk of eye diseases and retinal detachment as you age, which can also decrease your eye-related healthcare expenses. As an adult, you understand the costs involved when you or someone in your family develops a medical issue. There are the exams, treatment, prescription medications, possible hospital stays and surgery.

When it comes to your eye health, you not only have these expenses to worry about, but the maintenance costs as well. Glasses may last for a while, but they can easily get broken or lost and the higher your prescription is, the more expensive it becomes to purchase new glasses. Contact lenses also cost more depending on the condition of your eyes. If you have astigmatism or need multifocal contacts, you will end up paying more per box.

Should you develop an eye disease such as macular degeneration, you could pay as much as $1,500 for a single injection to slow the progression of the disease. One patient we know already had to have about sixty injections, and he will need to continue having them. Surgery to correct a retinal detachment is typically about $10,000, which doesn't include possible hospital stays, follow-up exams, or medications. Glaucoma surgery runs between $2,000 to $5,000, but should you choose a non-surgical method of treatment, it can cost as much as $2,000 a year for the rest of your life.

Since a vast number of people in this country don't have vision insurance, or if they do, it is grossly inadequate, who is going to pay all of these expenses? Even if you are lucky enough to have perfect vision, your insurance premiums help pay for everyone's medical care. Ortho-K lenses may seem expensive when compared to the cost of traditional corrective lenses, but when you weigh the cost against the financial benefits of reduced risk, you will discover that Ortho-K lenses are well worth it.

In addition to the decreased risk and reduced costs, adults can also benefit personally and socially from Ortho-K lenses. While most of the studies on self-perception and poor vision have been conducted on children, it can also affect adults. The impact glasses can have on self-perception does not necessarily go away as an individual ages. The individuals may get more used to wearing glasses over time but will likely continue to view themselves as they always had with glasses.

As eye doctors, we have had the pleasure of working with many adult patients who were fit with Ortho-K lenses, and the impact on their personalities from before their vision was corrected to after can be overwhelming. It is not uncommon to see normally shy and reserved adults become more outgoing. By giving them the freedom of clear vision, we have eliminated a source of stress from their lives so they can focus on other things.

With all these benefits, going with Ortho-K lenses to control your myopia seems like an easy choice. However, when making any decision about your eye health, it is important to weigh all the facts. Below, we have listed some questions you may want to ask yourself to determine if Ortho-K is right for you.

Do you struggle with wearing contacts due to seasonal or ongoing allergies?

Seasonal and year-round allergies can often lead to dry and itchy eyes. Many of my patients who deal with allergies may go weeks or sometimes months each year without wearing their contacts because the irritation is just too much. Their eyes are too itchy and the contacts only make things more uncomfortable. They are forced to wear their glasses, but then they have to deal with the inconvenience that comes with glasses, such as having them slip, fog up, or get lost. They also have to constantly remove their glasses to rub their eyes or put in eye drops.

Ortho-K lenses offer an enormous benefit to adults who suffer from seasonal or ongoing allergies. While they can't eliminate the allergies or the dry, itchy eyes, they can give you the freedom to go all day without the need for corrective lenses. You won't have to worry about contacts irritating your eyes, or your glasses getting in your way. Additionally, wearing Ortho-K lenses only at night means that the majority of the time spent wearing them your eyes are closed, minimizing the feeling of irritation and itchiness.

> *Wearing contacts at night, instead of in the day, is so great. I no longer have bloodshot, tearing eyes from dust or dryness. – Mary J.*

Do you suffer from dry eye?

Dry eye can be a serious problem that requires the ongoing use of medicated drops. Since most prescription eye drops cannot be used with contacts, this can prevent you from being able to wear contacts during the day. Dealing with constant eye irritation is bad enough, but having to change your daily routine or lifestyle to accommodate for glasses or contacts can be even more frustrating. Ortho-K lenses provide clear vision with the naked eye, so you can focus on treating your dry eye instead of dealing with the hassles of corrective lenses.

> *I have been a glasses and contact wearer for several years. I also frequently suffer from dry eyes. When my doctor suggested putting the Ortho-K lenses on me, I was willing to give them a try. They have been the most freeing process for me. No more contacts or glasses during the day and wearing them only when sleeping is perfect. My vision is good all day for reading, computer work, and driving. I'm so glad I took my doctor's advice. – Chris C.*

Are you tired of getting debris on your contacts or having them slip out of place while doing something?

If you've worn contacts for any length of time, you understand the instant irritation and discomfort you feel when an eyelash or bit of debris gets stuck to your lens. There are likely times when your eye has watered so much from something being in your eye that you can't even see clearly. Sometimes it's hard to get your eye to stay open long enough to get your contact out of your eye, and when you do, your eye is red and irritated for the rest of the day. You can't comfortably put your contact back in your eye because it is so irritated. Should this happen at work or while driving, it can not only be frustrating but dangerous. Even if you are just out with friends, playing with your kids, or just trying to relax and watch television, there is never a good time to have to deal with something stuck to your contact lens.

It can be just as frustrating to have your contact slip out of place or out of your eye completely. You are left with only one good eye while you fish around in the other eye for the out-of-place lens or scour the floor for where it might have dropped. Those nearly invisible tiny lenses can be quite challenging to find. Even if you do find it, you need to be somewhere where you can properly clean your hands and the lens before you put it back in.

One of the many benefits of Ortho-K is that it completely eliminates this frustration. You have the freedom to go about your day free from worry about your vision. The new shape of the cornea, which provides clear vision, also lasts longer than a day, so even if you accidentally drop your Ortho-K lens at night, you will still have clear vision to see what you are doing.

Do you enjoy sports, working out, hiking, skiing, or other outdoor activities?

It really doesn't matter what kinds of outdoor activities you are into. If you are an active person, you understand what a hindrance bad vision can be. The reliance on corrective lenses can create situations where you are more easily distracted and can't fully enjoy yourself.

Nobody enjoys losing a contact, especially when you are out in the woods hiking or on a snowy mountaintop skiing. Since it's not safe to wear contacts in water, your only option is to wear your glasses, but they can easily get lost when out kayaking or jet skiing. It's not only frustrating; it's costly. Not to mention, if you have to return home without your corrective lenses, you're putting yourself and others at risk by driving with uncorrected vision.

Ortho-K lenses are only worn at night, so you can enjoy perfect or near-perfect vision during the day without having to worry about breaking or losing your corrective lenses during recreational activities.

> *I can see clearly without any glasses! This has led to much more freedom with the hobbies I have – hiking, motorcycling, rock-climbing, etc. I can now wear sunglasses specific to these sports which give me much more protection and freedom. I also find that my face is much cooler without having to wear glasses all the time. In Arizona, that makes a huge difference. Additionally, it really makes watching TV and relaxing on the couch so much easier without a set of glasses to get in the way. There were times when the glasses would hurt my face or get broken depending on what I was doing. That doesn't happen anymore. For me, it's all about the freedom and flexibility that not having to wear prescription glasses brings. I really enjoy my Ortho-K lenses. – Juanita C.*

Have you ever wanted to try scuba diving or snorkeling?

Perhaps you've thought about going snorkeling or scuba diving while on vacation before, but you quickly gave up the idea due to your vision. It can be cumbersome trying to fit scuba goggles over your glasses. You might think wearing contacts would solve that problem, but wearing contacts in water, especially the ocean, increases your risk of getting eye infections. The last thing you want to worry about when on vacation is an eye infection.

Snorkeling and scuba diving are just two examples. There are so many other vacation activities that you may not be able to fully appreciate because of your poor vision. Traveling and sightseeing can be so much more fun and fulfilling when you see everything clearly. Eliminating the need for corrective lenses means you can enjoy your vacation without worrying about what to do if you lose or break your corrective lenses.

Ortho-K lenses allow you to wear sunglasses when it is sunny and still see perfectly. You can wear goggles when snorkeling, skydiving, parasailing, and jet skiing. There is no limit to what you can do and experience better and clearer with Ortho-K.

I have noticed that I can see much clearer without worrying about my glasses. I love seeing clearly while swimming and being able to see without a frame. Anyone who has any level of near-sightedness should use this system. They will be amazed at how clearly they can see without glasses. – Shona D.

Do you want to be able to see when you wake up during the night?

While there is currently nothing that will allow you to see in the dark aside from night-vision goggles, being able to see clearly can make a huge difference when navigating your surroundings in the dark. Many of my patients complain to me that their vision is so bad they have to put their glasses on just to go to the bathroom in the middle of the night. No one wants to be that dependent on corrective lenses. True freedom means being able to get up and go to the bathroom, get a drink of water, or check on your children in the middle of the night without needing your glasses.

Even though Ortho-K lenses are worn at night, you still have perfect vision while they are in. If you wake up, you will be able to see clearly as you move around your house.

I think it's very cool that I don't have to wake up and put on glasses. It also improved my piano and ballet. Thanks! – Lucy L.

Do you have or want a job that requires prefect vision?

Many jobs require or rely heavily on perfect or near-perfect vision. These professions include airline pilots, police officers, firemen, athletes, umpires, and some military positions such as Air Force pilots. Even as eye doctors, we found it frustrating trying to conduct eye exams with glasses on. We need to be able to look through a bioscope and back up again while still seeing perfectly. Constantly adjusting and removing our glasses was an inconvenience not only for us, but for our patients as well.

Even if a job doesn't require perfect vision, there are plenty that are simply easier to do without the hassle of corrective lenses. For example, being a chef is easier when you no longer have to deal with the worry of contacts or glasses in a hot kitchen. A photographer or any other profession where you have to look through a scope or viewfinder is easier without the headache of glasses. Who wants to constantly have to adjust their glasses while working on a road crew or building a house? With any construction or manufacturing job, there is an enormous amount of debris that can get in your eyes, which is why they typically require the use of safety goggles. However, it can be very uncomfortable to where safety goggles over glasses.

Ortho-K lenses eliminate these concerns by getting rid of the need for corrective lenses. They provide crisp, clear vision that lasts all day, so you can tackle anything your job throws your way.

> *Now, I can see clearly without glasses or contacts and I don't have to strain my eyes to see. – Grace M.*

Do you dislike contacts?

Obviously, daily soft contacts eliminate the hassle of wearing glasses. However, they come with their own host of problems, from eye irritation to eye infections. And forget about using them in water. The microbes in even your tap water can get trapped against your eye by soft contacts and can lead to eye infections.

If you have an allergy, or if something gets stuck to your lens, you may have to constantly adjust them or take them out several times throughout the day. They can also slip out of place fairly easily or even fall out of your eye completely. Depending on when and where that happens, it can be a serious hassle, not to mention it can even be dangerous if your contact slips out while you are driving.

Having to keep track of how many days you've been wearing your contacts adds yet another layer of frustration. If you wear them too long, it can increase your chances of eye irritation and infection. Dailies, soft contacts you wear for a day and then throw away, are convenient but more expensive than bi-weekly or monthly contacts. Dailies are also not suitable for some eye conditions, such as high astigmatism. Should you run out of contacts, you are stuck wearing your glasses until you can get more. Depending on your prescription, it can take up to a week from the time you order them to receive your new contacts.

Whatever the reason you don't like contact lenses, Ortho-K can eliminate your concerns. While they are contact lenses as well, you wear them while you are asleep, so you don't even feel them. Additionally, because you are sleeping when you have them in, you don't have to worry about them slipping out of place.

> *After a week of getting comfortable with my new Ortho-K lenses, I completely fell in love with them. It feels amazing to see clearly while at summer pool parties and never have to worry about having a contact pop out in the middle of a math test. I also don't have to worry about taking contacts out before a nap or spend time searching for misplaced glasses. Simply putting these lenses in before bed and waking up with perfect vision makes them incredibly convenient and easy. Now, I have been wearing them for over five years. They have made me more confident in both how I see and look. I definitely recommend Ortho-K lenses! – Emily K.*

Do you dislike wearing glasses?

Glasses have been around since the thirteenth century in one form or another, and while they may have been the standard for correcting poor vision until now, there are many people who don't like wearing glasses. Perhaps they don't like the way glasses feel on their face or the way they look in them. Glasses can leave red marks or indentations on your nose and around your ears. They can also be particularly irritating if you are sweating from working outside, exercising, or playing a sport as they can slip off your nose.

Having your glasses slip down can be especially frustrating if you have a job that requires you to constantly look up and down or be frequently bent over. No one wants to have to adjust their glasses every time they move their head. Bifocals can make this even worse since you have to constantly move your glasses around to line the lens up with what you are trying to see. You might find yourself giving up entirely and just take your glasses off everytime you need to read something.

Bending or breaking your glasses is also a major concern. Many people have active jobs that often result in their glasses being bent or broken. It is not uncommon to see someone who works in a manufacturing or labor position with bent, taped, or wired-together glasses. They break them so often that it typically isn't worth getting the glasses fixed every time. Having your glasses get scratched can also be extremely irritating. Any imperfection on the lens can impact your ability to see clearly. Protective glasses, which are less likely to bend, break, or get scratched, can be purchased, but they are generally more expensive. However, no glasses are indestructible.

For many people, glasses have become a deterrent. They avoid water activities or snow sports for fear of losing their glasses. They shy away from participating in most other sports as well, concerned they might break their glasses. In the summertime, glasses pose yet another problem. Unless you have prescription sunglasses, it is hard to protect your eyes from UV rays, yet doing so is important for the overall health of your eyes. UV rays can still cause damage to your eyes, even on cloudy days or during the winter. However, prescription sunglasses can be expensive. You can switch to wearing contacts, but as mentioned earlier, they come with their own set of concerns.

Ortho-K lenses offer you freedom from both glasses and contacts. Regardless of what your day has in store, you can handle it all with crisp, clear vision.

> *I've been wearing overnight contact lenses for fifteen years. This system is the way to go. It makes correcting your vision easy and convenient. I encourage anyone who is not happy with having to wear daytime contacts or glasses to check out this system. Since I am older, many times people have asked, "Don't you need glasses to read or see at a distance?" I just let them in on my little secret and recommend Ortho-K lenses. Now, I only have to wear them every other night. - Carolyn A.*

Are you interested in laser eye surgery, but concerned about the risks?

Over the last decade or so, LASIK surgery has gotten a lot of attention, which has led to more and more people asking their eye doctors if LASIK is right for them. Just as with any elective surgery, there are risks involved. Even if you are an ideal candidate for this procedure, and your chances of risk are low, you still need to be willing to accept that the worst case scenario may happen to you.

The risks associated with Ortho-K are significantly less. There is a risk of eye infection, but it is the same as with any overnight lens. However, that risk is minimal as long as you follow the proper care instructions.

One main advantage Ortho-K has over LASIK is that the results are not permanent. If you are unhappy with the results, or you find the lenses are uncomfortable to wear, you can simply stop using them and your vision will return to exactly as it was before starting Ortho-K.

A lot of the research conducted on Ortho-K in recent years has focused on children. That is, in part, because it is our children who will suffer from the future increased prevalence of eye diseases and retinal detachment. However, the benefits of Ortho-K are just as beneficial for adults as they are for children.

Even if your myopia has become severe, there is a solid chance Ortho-K lenses can correct your vision and stop the progression. People with a prescription of -6.00D are considered to have severe myopia, but just having a prescription over -5.00D increases your chances of developing myopic retinopathy by 5924 percent. It's never too late to get control of your myopia.

Many adults feel there is no point in changing now since they have been wearing glasses or contacts for years already. While change can be hard and may seem unnecessary when the status quo doesn't seem that bad, try to keep in mind that the progression of myopia is continuing to damage your eyes. You may not notice it happening or feel it, but it is true.

As your myopia progresses, your risk of developing potentially blinding eye diseases and retinal detachments increases. There are many people who feel that these eye diseases are just a part of growing older. However, it doesn't have to be that way. A lot of the elderly patients we see on a daily basis could have prevented their current vision problems by controlling their myopia.

The health of your eyes may seem less important when compared to other medical concerns like heart disease or cancer. However, the eyes are also quite literally the windows to the body. Your eyes are the only place where doctors can see your blood vessels without having to cut into you. Your doctor can detect high cholesterol and even leukemia through your eyes. Not only that, but just try to imagine your world without sight. Never being able to see your children's or grandchildren's faces again. Never being able to see the seasons change or gaze up at a beautiful starry sky. Maintaining the health of your eyes should be just as important as any other vital function and Ortho-K lenses can help you do that by trying to control the progression of myopia.

CHAPTER THIRTEEN

What to Expect When Getting Ortho-K Aligners

We have discussed all of the benefits of orthokeratology and why it's important to take control of your myopia now, but what can you expect when you actually get fit with overnight retainers? Many people feel anxious when experiencing something new, but knowing what to expect can help you feel calm as you move forward. Understanding the process will also help when it comes time to find the eye doctor who is right for you and your children.

As with any eye-care procedure, your doctor will start by giving you or your child a normal eye examination, checking for any problems or eye diseases you may be developing, such as glaucoma and cataracts. It is important that your doctor has an accurate assessment of your eyes' condition before beginning the Ortho-K process as these factors will help determine your level of treatment and can help predict the results. For example, if you are beginning to develop cataracts, your results with Ortho-K won't be as perfect as they would be for someone with mild to moderate myopia. This is due to the fact that the cataract (a clouding of the eye's natural lens) will continue to impede your vision regardless of the shape of your cornea. The only way to clear up vision lost from a cataract is through surgery. The optometrist will also determine your prescription. Since you already have myopia and likely needed contacts or glasses up until now, you probably already know what your prescription is. However, it may have changed since your last exam, so the doctor will still need to verify it. Once the exam is done, the doctor will take a digital map of the shape and topography of your eye. The surface of each cornea is as varied as fingerprints. No two are alike. With so many hills and valleys, the digital map is important for engineering Ortho-K lenses specific to you or your child. The more accurate the lenses, the better your results will be.

With the map completed, we can then use reverse geometry to create the interior shape of the lens for each eye. As mentioned in Chapter Nine, the interior shape is not only important for the actual process of reshaping the cornea (which gives you clearer vision), but it is also necessary so that the lens stays centered on the eye. Keeping it centered means more comfort and better results.

Before ordering your custom lenses, your doctor may have some sample lenses for you to try. Since Ortho-K lenses are rigid, they can take some getting used to for some patients, particularly if the patients were used to soft contacts. It is important to try the lenses out before ordering the custom ones, so you can decide if they are right for you. Using the sample lenses, you will then be taught how to place the aligner on your eye, how to remove it from your eye, and how to care for it. Placing the lenses on yours or your child's eyes may take some practice, especially if you are not use to touching your eye. For example, people who have worn soft contacts may be more comfortable learning how to place the lenses.

Regardless of how you may have been taught to care for your soft contacts, it is extremely important to follow your eye doctor's instructions on the proper care for your Ortho-K lenses. This is especially true for children. Not properly cleaning and caring for the contact lenses is the main cause for eye infections. Parents of young patients should pay attention to the doctor's instructions as well so that they can supervise their children until proper habits have been established, and the child can care for the lenses independently.

The lenses should be thoroughly cleaned each day and only with approved solutions. Your doctor will help you pick a contact solution that is right for you. Since there is a complex relationship between your eyes, the lenses, and the solutions with which they are cleaned and stored, using the wrong solution could not only be uncomfortable, but it could actually warp your Ortho-K lenses. It is for this reason that many eye drops are not approved for use with contacts. If your Ortho-K lenses become warped, they could be rendered ineffective, affecting how well you are able to see. Only use solutions or eye drops that have been recommended by your doctor. Should the recommended solution cause any itching or irritation, talk to your doctor before changing to a different one.

Equally important is to make sure your hands are clean and dry before touching your eyes or handling the aligners. As eye doctors, we recommend

What to Expect When Getting Ortho-K Aligners

Dear Dr. David Roth,

I would like to thank you for introducing me to Ortho-K (vision correction without surgery.. GMT). It has been a miracle, as a firefighter and as a rescue specialist for South Florida's Task Force 2, the demands on my vision are extraordinary. As a firefighter I work 24 hour shifts and for the last 8 yea...rs contacts where not cutting it. Dr Roth the true medical professional suggested I look into Ortho-K (vision correction without surgery..GMT). . Since then there are many lives that can thank him. I will never forget when he told me not to expect 20/20 especially with the rigors I put my body through. And I regret to tell you that I do not have 20/20; I have better. About 20/15 six hours after taking my lenses off. In January, Haiti experienced an earthquake that not only changed the life of many Haitians but also mine and a lot of my colleagues on South Florida's Task Force 2. We were there 48 hours after the ground shook and did not stop till we left 14 days later. During my tour there my first 80 hours where without much rest. I really had no time to worry about my eyes sorry Dr Roth. My vision was tested and after daily medical assessments, I was still cleared with 20/40 vision with much amazement from our physician. After the fourth day on the island I got to rest for 4 hours I put in my Ortho-K lenses and wore them through our briefing for a total of 5 hours. And went to work for another 36 hours with little breaks lasting about 30 min each. Did that day in and day out till we got back and have worn them every night since. All I can say is that I can't express in words what I owe Dr Roth for what he has done for me and my family but thank you and he has a personal media here with me. There is a joke in the fire service and it is, there are many ways to spread good or bad news, Television, telephone, telegraph, and tell a fireman. And all I got to say, is if you're thinking about it just do it you won't regret anything about it.

Thank you,
Oscar

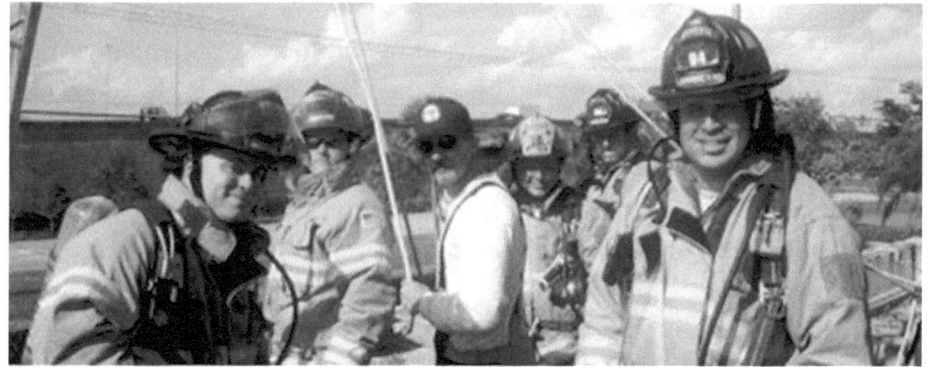

using mild, unscented dish soap to wash your hands, and that you dry them with a clean lint-free towel. Even if your hands are clean, touching your eyes or the aligners with wet hands can transfer any microbes from your tap water to your eyes. Following proper care instructions will dramatically reduce and likely eliminate the risk of developing an eye infection.

As mentioned in previous chapters, there were several cases of children in China who used Ortho-K lenses and developed severe eye infections. At first, the lenses were blamed, and many people, both within the eye-care community and not, believed they were unsafe to use. However, after repeated investigations into the situation, it was determined that the children may not have received proper care instructions. The infections were likely a result of the lenses not being properly cleaned each day, with some patients simply rinsing them under tap water to clean them. Other patients are believed to have worn their lenses during the day as opposed to at night. Additional factors that were examined during the investigations were the type of material used in the lenses and the knowledge and training of the providers.

After you or your child has been thoroughly examined, the proper prescription has been measured, and the topography of your cornea has been mapped, your doctor can proceed with ordering your custom aligners. Each aligner is made to perfectly fit a patient's eye. Since each of your eyes is different, the aligners will also be different, meaning the lenses will not be interchangeable. You will receive an aligner specifically made for your right eye and one for your left eye. This custom engineering improves the comfort and success of the lenses.

Once the aligners are ready, you will return for an evaluation appointment where the custom lenses are placed in your eyes for the first time. Your orthokeratologist will then take several measurements to ensure they are the right fit. Before leaving your doctor's office, you will have to practice to make sure you can place and remove the lenses from yours or your child's eyes.

It has been our experience that it isn't until children are about ten years old that they really start to successfully insert their own aligners. However, every child is different. We have had patients as young as six who can do it themselves, as well as patients who are older than ten who still need help from their parents. The important thing is that parents gauge their child's ability for themselves and work with their child until he or she can properly insert and remove the lenses on their own.

The aligners will likely feel weird at first. A lot of people find rigid contacts, whether day- or nighttime-use lenses, to take some getting used to when they first start wearing them. This is one of the reasons why soft contacts are the more popular choice. However, as mentioned in previous chapters, using soft contacts may actually increase your risk of progressive myopia.

While some people find that they can feel the aligners at first, it is not actually the sensation of the lens on their eyeball that they are feeling. Instead, it is their eyelids brushing the edge of the lens. Whenever patients complain about how the lenses feel, we have them try closing their eyes, and then ask them to tell us how the lenses feel now. Once their eyes are closed, they can barely feel the lenses at all. Since these lenses are only worn while you are sleeping, there is no need for concern about discomfort.

Depending on your orthokeratologist and the level of treatment required, you will be instructed to wear the aligners each night for up to three weeks. This will give you a chance to not only get used to placing, removing, and cleaning them, but to how they feel as well. When you return for your follow-up visit, your optometrist will assess the improvements to your vision. This is also a good opportunity to ask any questions you might have.

Typically, our patients experience a 30 to 50 percent improvement in their vision after just one night of wear. They continue to have as much as a 50 percent improvement each consecutive night until they experience perfect or near-perfect daytime vision. The impact of the overnight lenses lasts the entire day, sometimes longer, so you will not need to wear any form of corrective lens during the day.

We recommend patients come back for follow-up appointments after the first week, and then after one month, three months, six months and finally twelve months. At the one-year check-up, we take more measurements to make a new set of lenses. Since the aligners have done their job by this point, in *aligning* the cornea, the new lenses will act as retainers. Similar to dental retainers, these lenses are designed to keep the corneas in the desired shape. As mentioned in previous chapters, the effects of Ortho-K lenses are completely reversible. Even if you have been wearing the retainers for forty years, your eyes will still go back to the way they were before you started Ortho-K should you stop wearing the lenses. That is why continuing to wear them each night is imperative if you want to maintain crisp, clear vision.

Regardless of whether they are aligners or retainers, each set of lenses is only good for about a year. Even with proper care and cleaning, the lenses can build up layers of residue from daily handling. This build-up is practically invisible to the naked eye, but it can increase the risk of eye infections. There is also the possibility of scratches developing due to the necessary daily handling and cleaning. Even if the lenses look and feel normal, it is important to get new retainers made each year.

When considering this option of myopia control, it is important to not simply choose the cheapest one. Overnight lenses are going to be more expensive than traditional glasses or contacts. However, the cost is significantly less than the cost of treatment or surgery for eye diseases or retinal detachment. So, consider the expense as an investment in the current and future health of yours or your child's eyes.

A doctor who is just starting out with Ortho-K may offer reduced rates to attract new customers, but it is usually a good indication of the doctor's confidence in his or her ability. Even now, there are relatively few optometrists and ophthalmologists who specialize in overnight lenses. Out of the some forty-thousand eye-care professionals in this country, there are probably fewer than five hundred who specialize in orthokeratology.

This is why it is so important to ask questions and do research before choosing a doctor. In the following chapter, we will discuss what questions to ask, as well as what things to look for and consider when choosing which orthokeratologist is right for you.

While the vast majority of our patients have found success, there is a small percentage who have not. Worldwide, over one million patients have been successfully fit with Ortho-K lenses. However, not everyone is the best candidate. There are many factors that make someone a poor candidate for Ortho-K, including heredity, scar tissue from surgeries, and overall health. Although the rate of success is very high, it is important to understand that Ortho-K does not work for every single patient.

Since there is currently no way to maintain your improved vision except through the use of the retainers, you will need to continue wearing them each night for the rest of your life. Just like brushing your teeth, putting your retainers in will become part of your nighttime routine. This may seem like a huge commitment, but when compared to the risks of progressive myopia, that commitment is relatively small. Ortho-K lenses offer many long-term benefits beyond simply getting rid of your need for glasses or contacts. As long as you continue wearing your overnight lenses, you will be able to keep your vision stable and possibly decrease your risk of potentially blinding eye diseases and retinal detachment. Not only that, but you will be able to continue to enjoy the freedom of seeing without glasses.

CHAPTER FOURTEEN

Choosing a Doctor for Ortho-K

With so few optometrists and ophthalmologists in this country currently offering Ortho-K, it may seem like a daunting task to find a doctor, let alone one with the experience to provide the level of treatment you or your child needs. However, don't throw in the towel just yet. By doing a little bit of leg-work and research, you can find the doctor who is right for you or your child.

Each year, the Orthokeratology Academy of America (OAA) and other orthokeratology associations host conferences where doctors can come together to share new ideas and best practices. They also offer beginner boot-camp sessions on Ortho-K for any attending optometrist or ophthalmologist interested in learning more about this technology and how they can begin offering it in their practice. These boot camps usually attract anywhere between seventy to two hundred new doctors every time.

While this turnout is promising, doctors still have to overcome the traditional mindset within the eye-care community that laser surgery is the way to go when correcting refractive errors. Since eye surgery has been around longer than Ortho-K and had the backing of laser manufacturers, ophthalmologists have been ingrained to think that reshaping the cornea with invasive lasers is better than reshaping it non-invasively with rigid contacts. However, it is our sincere hope that more doctors will come to embrace this technology and help us in the fight against the myopia epidemic.

That being said, just because a doctor says he or she offers Ortho-K doesn't make him or her the right doctor for you. You will want to check into the doctors, as well as their practice, to make sure they are affordable, helpful, knowledgeable, and pleasant. That is why doing a bit a research before scheduling a consultation is so important.

Obviously, a personal recommendation from someone you trust is the preferred way to find a specialty doctor. However, if you don't have someone to offer a recommendation, you shouldn't let that stop you. Your regular eye doctor or family physician may be able to give you a recommendation. There is also the option of contacting one of the contributing doctors of this book. Each one is highly skilled, with years of experience fitting patients with Ortho-K. If they are not located in your area, they may be able to recommend a doctor who is.

The Internet is another way you can find orthokeratologists in your area. While these doctors may not come with a personal recommendation, you can check out their websites for testimonials and customer reviews. If you find negative reviews online, don't be afraid to ask the doctor about them. The review may have been left by a patient who was mad that the process didn't work, which doesn't necessarily reflect on the quality of the care provided.

You can usually find the doctor's biography on the website as well, along with information about the doctor's education, training, and experience. If this information is not available through the website, you should ask for printed copies of it when contacting the office. This should give you a good starting point from which you can narrow down the list of candidates.

Even though orthokeratology has been around for more than four decades, many people have never heard of this technology before, so many patients approach Ortho-K with a wide range of questions and concerns. While we hope we have addressed many of your questions and concerns in this book, identifying what concerns you *do* have will help you when choosing a doctor. Creating a list of questions and concerns can act as a guide so you will know exactly what you are looking for. Is cost a priority for you? Or maybe comfort level? Whatever your concerns, identifying them will help you know which questions to ask when the time comes.

Some of the common concerns and fears I have come across with my patients are:

- Fear of trying something new
- Concern that the lenses will interfere with their normal activities
- Concern that the lenses will hurt or be uncomfortable
- Concern that their family will be critical of their decision to try something they have never heard of
- Fear they won't be able to afford the retainers long-term
- Concern over finding a doctor who is right for them

Choosing a Doctor for Ortho-K

Once you have identified what concerns you still have and what your treatment priorities are, you can start calling the offices on your list. Believe me, you can tell a lot about a doctor's practice simply by calling, even if you only get to speak with the receptionist. When choosing a practice, keep in mind that you won't just be dealing with the doctor. You will likely have to deal with the doctor's staff, his or her assistants, billing personnel, and receptionists, which can make your experience either a positive or a negative one.

Here is a list of things to ask yourself when calling a doctor's practice for the first time:
- Was the call answered in no more than four rings?
- Did you get a busy signal?
- Were you immediately placed on hold, and if so, for how long?
- Were you greeted in a friendly, warm manner? Or did you feel interrupted and/or like you were bothering the person answering the phone?
- Was the person answering the phone helpful and knowledgeable? Was it apparent that this person was trained to understand Ortho-K and answer general questions?
- If you asked a question that person couldn't answer, were you immediately connected with someone who could answer it? Were you offered additional material to help you make your decision, such as offering to mail you a brochure or pamphlet? Or were you directed to the office's website? If they didn't have any additional information available, it may be a sign that the office either hadn't been offering Ortho-K for very long, or they haven't had a lot of Ortho-K patients.

If your answers to these questions were positive, your next step would be to schedule a consultation. However, if more than one answer was negative, or you just got an overall bad impression when talking to that office, hang up and move on to the next office on your list. Your time is valuable, and you shouldn't waste it by scheduling a consultation with an office that is probably not right for you.

If you did schedule a consultation:
- Were you offered multiple appointment options?
- Were your appointment date and time confirmed?
- Did the person you were talking to give you his or her name and the names of other staff members you could ask for if you called back with questions?
- Were you informed of any consultation fees upfront?

- If you asked about fees, were you provided with useful information? While the exact amount can only be determined after your consultation as it depends on a number of factors, the person you were speaking with should be able to provide you with an estimated price range.
- Did the person you were talking to ask you when the best time to reach you is and if you have a preferred phone number? This is a good indication that they are just as interested in working with you as you are in working with them.

Once you have scheduled consultations with your preferred candidates, you might want to consider making up a list of questions to bring with you. In the October 2003 issue of *Cosmetic Surgery News*, Susan Fontana advised, "The written list is extremely important because it is very easy to feel intimidated and forget what you want to ask." In a way, your consultation is kind of like a job interview, where you evaluate the doctor before deciding whether to *hire* him or her for the job. Just as an employer has a list of questions for their prospective employee, so too should you have a list of question to ask your prospective doctor.

Below, I have listed the questions I recommend every patient ask each of their prospective doctors.

1. Is the doctor board-certified? If so, which board are they certified with? Keep in mind, however, that even if they are board-certified, it doesn't mean they are better at the procedure.
2. Which type of topographer does the doctor use? If the doctor says he or she is not using a topographer then he or she probably isn't a doctor you want to work with. The only way to accurately map the shape of your cornea so that Ortho-K lenses can be custom designed for you is by using a topographer.
3. Does the doctor get any referrals from other doctors for this procedure? If so, how many referrals do they typically get per month?
4. How many patients does the doctor typically see per month for this procedure? If they usually fit fewer than five new patients per month, they probably don't have the level of experience you are looking for.
5. When was the last time the doctor fitted a new patient? If it was more than a month prior, again, this doctor probably doesn't have much experience.

6. How many Ortho-K patients is the doctor currently working with? Aligners are typically worn for about a year before the patient transitions to retainers, so the doctor continues to work with these patients during that time. A doctor currently working with thirty patients is going to have more overall experience than a doctor currently working with two.
7. How much of the doctor's practice is dedicated to Ortho-K? If Ortho-K seems like an afterthought at that doctor's office, it probably is, which means they likely don't fit very many new patients.
8. How long has the doctor been offering Ortho-K? Even if the doctor has been offering the procedure for a long time, if they don't regularly fit new patients, their level of experience is probably low.
9. What is the doctor's success rate? Even if the doctor has fit more than a thousand patients with Ortho-K lenses, if their success rate is only one in two (or 50 percent), you probably don't want to trust them with your eyes. Quantity does not equal quality.
10. How many appointments are typically required during the first year of treatment? What about the second year?
11. How long does the doctor estimate it will be until you are able to see clearly enough to drive or play sports without corrective lenses? Depending on your original prescription, you should notice a difference after the first night of wearing the lenses. The amount of time it takes your eyesight to be clear enough to drive or play sports without corrective lenses can take anywhere from one night to a couple of weeks, depending on how severe your myopia was to begin with.
12. Will the doctor provide you with an itemized quote of costs? In addition to the cost of lenses, it is important to know what other fees are involved. Ortho-K lenses can cost anywhere from $1,500 to $5,000, depending on the patient's eye condition and the level of treatment required. Additional costs may include the exams, cleaning solution, gels, drops, storage cases for the lenses, replacement lenses, and fittings.
13. Does their office offer any kind of financing? If so, what are the terms of the financing? Similar to orthodontists, many eye doctors set their patients up on a monthly payment plan to make the cost more feasible.

14. Should you be unhappy with your results, does the doctor's office offer any refunds? If so, how many refunds did they give out in the last year? What are the terms of the refund? Refunds can vary greatly from one doctor to the next, so it is important to understand that doctor's policy prior to having your custom lenses made.
15. Which procedure does the doctor perform most frequently?
16. Is additional information, such as brochures or pamphlets, given at the consultation to take home and study?
17. How long has the doctor's staff been employed at that office? Are they experienced enough to answer questions if the doctor is not available?
18. How many doctors in office are trained in Ortho-K? This is important as you want to make sure there will always be a doctor available if you need to come in for an emergency visit.
19. Does the doctor have any patient consultants? These are people who have been through the process and can offer a firsthand account of the experience. If not, do they have patient testimonials? Sometimes doctors will have patient testimonials up on their website, but if not, make sure to ask about them at the consultation. If the doctor can't provide any testimonials, it is probably a sign they haven't been offering this procedure very long.
20. Is the doctor's biography available on their website? As I mentioned earlier, this can provide valuable information about the doctor's training and experience. If their bio is not up on their website, ask for a printed copy at the consultation.
21. Has the doctor written books or medical journal articles on Ortho-K? While it is certainly not necessary that they have, it is a good indication they have extensive knowledge about this procedure.
22. Has the doctor taught other doctors his methods? Again, it is not necessary for every doctor you interview to be a teacher as well, but knowing the doctor is experienced enough to be training other doctors can help ease your concerns.
23. What are the doctor's recommendations for long-term success with Ortho-K? If any recommendation seems outlandish, it is a good indication the doctor is probably still unfamiliar with this procedure.
24. How often does the doctor recommend the lenses be replaced? I recommend all of my patients get new lenses every year. The retainers can warp from daily cleaning and get scratched from proteins building

up on the lenses, increasing the risk of eye infections and irritation. If the doctor tells you the lenses can last longer than a year, be skeptical.

25. Does the doctor offer daytime lenses/retainers for patients who don't want to wear them while sleeping? Ortho-K lenses are designed for nighttime use to increase patient comfort. However, depending on their lifestyle, some patients prefer daytime lenses.
26. Does the doctor have the capacity to create custom lenses for treating special conditions? Or are the treatment lenses out of a kit? Some types of orthokeratology lenses are a one-size-fits-all, which in actuality really only work for one type or shape of eye. Since everyone's eyes are shaped differently, trying to fit every patient with the same lens can not only cause eye irritation, but is the main reason some patients don't have success.
27. Ask the doctor to list off their pros and cons of Ortho-K.
28. Ask the doctor about any risks involved or if there are any side effects. We have covered the risks of Ortho-K in previous chapters but it is still a good idea to ask your prospective doctor, in the event he or she has noticed side effects in some of his or her patients. It may be a sign the doctor is not giving adequate care instructions or proper fittings.
29. Ask the doctor about proper care and maintenance. What type of contact solution does he or she recommend?
30. How many follow-up appointments does the doctor require? How long can you expect each appointment to take? I typically have my patients return for follow-up appointments at one week, one month, three months, six months, and twelve months. The length of each appointment depends on the individual patient's eye condition and how they are responding to the lenses.
31. How are the lenses designed for each patient? Does the doctor take measurements of each eye? What equipment does he or she use? It is extremely difficult to get the correct interior shape of the lens without making a digital map of the cornea's surface. If the doctor does not have the proper equipment to take these measurements, it is a good indication they are not familiar with this procedure. Doctors who don't have much experience or knowledge may be offering one-size-fits-all Ortho-K lenses, and likely have a lower success rate.
32. Is the doctor comfortable with working on more than one custom lens design? As no two eyes are alike, each lens needs

to be specifically engineered for each of your eyes. If the doctor is not comfortable with engineering each lens, you are not going to get lenses made specifically for your eyes, which may cause discomfort and hinder your results.

33. How would you benefit from choosing this doctor? What makes them different from other doctors you have interviewed?
34. How does the doctor determine if children can wear Ortho-K lenses? What does he or she recommend are your other options for stabilizing your child's eyes if your child is not a good candidate for Ortho-K?
35. Are the lenses uncomfortable? How long does it typically take until patients get used to the lenses?
36. Upon agreeing to move forward with the procedure, is there a contract that needs to be signed, ensuring the doctor is as committed to the arrangement as you are?

In addition to making a list of questions to ask during your consultation, you may want to write down any and all symptoms you are currently experiencing as well. Make sure to list everything, even if the symptom doesn't pertain to your eyes. It is also a good idea to make a list of any medications you are taking, as some medications can affect your eye health. You might consider bringing a family member or friend with you to your consultation, someone whose opinion you respect, as they can offer a different perspective on the interview.

Once you have met with each of your prospective doctors, assess how each consultation went. Which doctors took the time to listen to and clearly answer your questions? Did they explain things in terms you could understand? Which practices kept your consultation to your appointed time and which offices made you wait? Did you feel pressured at any time during the consultation? Did the doctor try to talk you out of using Ortho-K lenses? Maybe they tried to pressure you into signing up for Ortho-K right then and there. Did the doctor or office staff seem annoyed or hurried? Did a financial manager explain the costs and financing options for you?

Here, Dr. Mark Page shares his own experiences with orthokeratology: Being an Ortho-K patient myself, I understand just how daunting choosing a doctor can be. I have been wearing retainers for more than twelve years now, and back when I first got fit with the lenses there were even fewer doctors offering Ortho-K. My vision had gotten so bad that it was beginning to impact my ability to do my job. I was constantly having to take my glasses off to look through the microscope during patient exams. At first, I contemplated getting LASIK, but I wasn't ready to accept the risks. Since LASIK eye surgery doesn't work for everyone, I was concerned that I would not only be risking my eyesight but my career as well.

This motivated me to look for another option. I did a great deal of research on my own, reading about twenty medical journals a month to keep up on the newest options and latest improvements in my field. Finally, I discovered orthokeratology. At the time, there were very few myopia control options available and even fewer optometrists who specialized in them.

I decided to try the lenses myself to see how they worked. CRT (Corneal Refractive Therapy) lenses were easily accessible as they were being made right down the road from his office. However, I soon discovered that they simply didn't work for everyone. CRT lenses are designed for people who have very round eyes, but not everyone's eyes are that shape. Some people have more oval or oblong-shaped eyes, yet any deviation from the perfectly round shape led to the patient experiencing less than ideal results. There was also a lack of vision improvement. Because CRT lenses are not designed for each patient's specific eye shape, the lenses don't always fit properly. Without a proper fit, the lens can't create a vacuum on the cornea to reshape it.

Temporarily forced to stop recommending CRT lenses to patients as it became too difficult to know if they would work or not, I started focusing on learning how to custom-make lenses myself. This allowed me to adjust the interior shape of the lenses based on the shape of each individual patient's eye. Some of my patients who did not find success with the CRT lenses returned, and I fitted them with my custom-made lenses. Each patient I fit with the new lenses had success, and their vision improved. I now use custom-made lenses for almost all of my patients. I call this line of custom lenses *Invisalens*.

Optometrists who are highly experienced with Ortho-K and are familiar with the process of creating the lenses are capable of engineering custom lenses based on each patient's needs and the shape of their eyes. While the success of Ortho-K lenses will vary based on several factors, including the patient's prescription, treatment goals, heredity, and overall health, choosing a doctor who can engineer custom lenses for you or your child is essential for success with Ortho-K. With a little bit of research and by following the steps outlined in this chapter, you can gain the confidence to select the doctor who is right for you or your child.

CHAPTER FIFTEEN

Here's to Your Eye Health!

With 85 percent of your total knowledge obtained through sight, your eyes are, without a doubt, your most precious sense. Color, shape, texture, distance, light, shadow—there are numerous things you can discern about an object just by seeing it. Your eyes also allow you to read, which makes the possibilities for learning almost limitless.

This is especially true for children. About 80 percent of all their learning is perceived through their eyes. So, just imagine what having a refractive error such as myopia can do to your child's education. Whether or not your child is currently myopic, protecting his or her eyes now will preserve their vision into the future.

Your eyes are one of the most complex organs in your body and have more than two million working parts that can process more than 36,000 pieces of information every hour. Directly connected to your brain, your eyes use up to 65 percent of the brain's neural pathways. Your eyes can also see the light of a single candle up to fourteen miles away if the conditions are right.

Your eyes never rest. While it's true that the muscles around your eyes and your eyelids need to rest, your actual eyeballs are always functioning at 100 percent of their ability, day or night. They are also the only place in your body where your blood vessels and arteries can be viewed without involving invasive techniques such as surgery. Because of this, your doctor can see signs of illnesses affecting other areas of your body through your eyes, including high cholesterol, heart disease, leukemia, and lung cancer.

Most people seem to think that an eye exam consists of simply checking for vision problems and providing a prescription for corrective lenses. However, your eye doctor can actually discern a lot about your overall health through your eyes. When cholesterol levels are elevated, the cholesterol can collect in a white ring around the cornea on the outside of the eyeball. Since high cholesterol is a major risk factor for heart disease, this white ring can be an indication that heart disease is developing. Leukemia, a cancer that affects blood cells, can be detected through the eyes due to the unique patterns of bleeding it can cause. Some patients with lung cancer can develop tumors in their eyes. In fact, about 8 percent of all skin cancer diagnoses are discovered on the eyelids.

Considering how precious your eyes are, one of the most important things you can do for yours or your child's sight is to get regular eye exams. There is a common misconception that only people with vision problems need to see an eye doctor. This is completely untrue. Just as you should go to a physician annually for a physical check-up, or to the dentist every six months for cleanings, you should see an eye doctor at least annually for an eye exam. Even if your vision is 20/20, it is important to get checked regularly for any developing eye diseases and, as mentioned earlier, your eye doctor may discover signs of other illnesses. Early detection is key when it comes to diagnosing disease, and it could save your life.

Numerous people have vision problems and they aren't even aware of them. Glaucoma is a perfect example. More than half of glaucoma patients don't actually know they have the disease. As mentioned in Chapter Two, glaucoma is when fluid pressure builds up in the eye, usually due to the blockage of the mesh framework bordering your iris. As this pressure increases, it puts strain on the optic nerve, potentially damaging it. If left untreated, glaucoma can lead to severe vision loss. Since glaucoma is usually painless most people don't realize they have the disease until they have some level of vision loss. However, if it is diagnosed early enough, the disease can be easily treated.

The same can be said for myopia. Some patients don't seek help from an eye doctor until their myopia has already progressed to moderate levels. They don't notice that they have an issue until they can no longer read the white board from the back of the classroom or read road signs until they are driving past them.

Myopia can be especially hard to notice in kids. Children typically don't understand that the blurriness they see is not normal, so they don't speak up. Approximately one in every four children has an undetected vision problem. Most public schools do offer eye exams, but the tests are usually inadequate, looking only for obvious refractive errors and sometimes color blindness. The best way to truly preserve yours and your child's eye health is through early detection by means of an annual exam.

Another misconception some patients have is that the stronger their prescription is, the faster their eyes will get worse. For this reason, we often get parents requesting that we under-prescribe their child's glasses or contacts. So, if the child's eyes are at a -2.00D, the parents would request that their glasses be at a -1.75D or -1.50D.

However, the opposite is true. Two separate studies have proven that patients who were under-prescribed on their corrective lenses actually had their myopia progress faster. Because the prescription is weaker than what is needed, the eyes have to strain to focus, causing the eyeball to stretch and elongate, which increases the myopia. As the patient's vision worsens, the prescription becomes even weaker, causing more eye strain and stretching, resulting in a downward spiral of worsening vision. If you opt to use corrective lenses, always get the correct prescription and have your eye doctor check your prescription at your annual eye exam.

While having a higher prescription doesn't cause your myopia to progress faster, it does increase your risk of developing eye diseases and retinal detachments. The odds of developing a retinal detachment if your prescription is -1.00D to -2.75D are 3.1 to 1. If your prescription is -9.00D to 14.75D, the odds ratio skyrockets to 44.2 to 1. To put that into perspective, if you have a -1.00D prescription you are three times more likely to develop a detached retina. If you have a -9.00D prescription, you are forty-four times more likely to develop a detached retina. As the odds increase, the chances of something bad happening also increase, just based on the strength of your prescription. This is why controlling yours or your child's myopia now is so important.

Some other misconceptions patients tend to have are that all eye doctors are the same, and that all corrective lenses are created equal. When it comes to eye doctors, there is a distinction between optometrists and ophthalmologists. While optometrists can examine, diagnose, and prescribe medications for patients, they cannot perform eye surgery, yet ophthalmologists can. There are also differences between state requirements of education and training, not to mention on-the-job experience. Just as every patient has different vision problems, every eye doctor has different levels of experience and skills, making choosing the right doctor for you so important.

Corrective lenses also differ depending on the material with which they are made, what treatment is applied, and what tools are used. While reading glasses can be purchased without a prescription from your local drugstore, the quality of those glasses is vastly inferior to the ones prescribed and ordered by your eye doctor. The difference between soft and rigid contact lenses can be equated to the difference between disposable cameras and digital ones. Like soft contacts, disposable cameras are cheap and convenient, but they don't offer the same level of quality a digital camera does.

The last misconception we often hear from patients is that you can improve your vision through eye exercises or hypnosis. While it is true that doing exercises can strengthen the muscles of your eyes, just as weight training does for your arms or legs, strengthening your eye muscles does nothing to improve your vision. Your eye muscles close and open your eyelid or move your eyeball around as you look in different directions, but your ability to see has to do with how light enters your eye. Whether you see clearly or not depends on how light is refracted against your retina. If there is a problem with the curvature of your cornea or your eye's natural lens, your vision will be impaired, both of which neither exercises nor hypnosis can correct. So, beware of companies or websites that claim they can teach you to see clearly through either of these methods. As eye doctors, each of us has had several patients who have actually worsened their vision by following these types of programs.

I urge all of my patients to think about theirs and their children's sight in the long term. Even if your current risk for eye disease is low, how might your lifestyle now affect your vision later in life? The Vision Council of America's (VCA) statistics state that more than ten million Americans suffer from vision problems related to too much time spent on electronic devices and computers. Other studies suggest that nutrition plays a role in eye health. The increased intake of sugar and processed carbohydrates in our diets, along with the decreased consumption of fresh fruits and vegetables, may be contributing to our country's vision problems. Making simple changes to your everyday lifestyle, such as applying the 20-20-20 rule mentioned in Chapter Seven and watching what foods you eat, can help preserve your eye health in the future.

Approximately eighty-six million Americans over the age of forty are affected by vision deficiencies, and that number is expected to nearly double in the next few decades. Currently, one in three adults over the age of fifty-five has an eye disease that impairs their vision. With the current prevalence of myopia, the number of people with eye diseases is projected to increase dramatically as the younger generations age. However, the prevalence of myopia is also expected to increase, making that number even larger.

Age-related macular degeneration is currently the leading cause of blindness in people over the age of fifty. It is a painless eye disease that causes permanent loss of central vision, and many adults don't even realize they have it until it is too late. Normally, macular degeneration can be attributed to a lifetime's worth of sun-exposure, which is why it is usually referred to as *age-related*. However, as our daily use of computers and electronic devices increases, we will start to see more cases of non-age-related macular degeneration.

As discussed in Chapter Five, exposure to the blue light emitted from modern electronic devices and computer monitors can damage the macula in much the same way UV rays from the sun do. However, for most of us it isn't feasible to simply stop using our computers. Websites like *lowbluelights.com* sell blue light-blocking glasses and filters that can be applied to your computer monitor and device screens. The yellow film reduces the amount of blue light that enters your eyes, preserving the health of your macula. There are also apps you can download such as *f.lux*, which changes the amount of light emitted from your display to mimic natural daytime light cycles.

While 88 percent of Americans know that extended sun exposure can cause skin cancer, fewer than 9 percent are aware that the sun can also harm and damage their eyes. Not only do the UV rays in sunlight damage the macula, but they can also damage the photoreceptors at the back of your eyes. Normally, these photoreceptors will regenerate over time, but cumulative sun exposure can damage them to the point that they will no longer be able to regenerate.

Sunlight exposure can also cause photoreceptor overload, which is when all of the pigment gets bleached out of your photoreceptors. If your photoreceptors become bleached by too much sunlight exposure during the day, that exposure can affect how well you see at night. This is why some pilots are not allowed to fly at night if they don't properly protect their eyes during the day. Using dark-tinted lenses, such as sunglasses, allows less light to enter your eye. Your eyes then become used to that level of light exposure, which can enhance your nighttime vision.

When not exposed to too much sunlight during the day, your eyes can actually adjust to fully dark conditions within about thirty minutes. However, studies suggest that as little as two to three hours of unprotected sunlight exposure can delay this adjustment for hours. For example, just ten consecutive days of full-sun exposure can decrease your nighttime visual clarity, contrast, and range by up to 50 percent.

To maximize your nighttime vision, we recommend always wearing sunglasses and hats when exposed to sunlight. When driving at night, try dimming your dash lights. Your car's interior dimmer is designed to be adjusted, allowing you to make the light inside the cabin just bright enough for the instruments on your dash to remain safely legible. Just as it is hard to see outside at night from a lit room, the dimmer the interior light, the better your visibility will be.

When choosing sunglasses, be careful of misleading labels. Unlike Australia, the United States has no regulations on the UV protection of sunglasses, so going by what the labels say doesn't mean that is what you are getting. Approximately 80 percent of manufactured sunglasses are made from inferior acrylic material as well and account for most of the consumer complaints eye doctors receive of strain and headaches.

Do some research before wasting your money on inadequate sunglasses. Try to find ones with HEV (high-energy visible) polarized lenses. Sunglasses with HEV polarized lenses can reduce glare and provide the best possible outdoor vision. You can also consider taking your sunglasses in to have your eye doctor test them. Some optometrists have special equipment which can read the UV protection levels of lenses.

Remember, sunlight damage is cumulative, so protecting yours and your child's eyes from sun exposure now is extremely important for your future eye health. Studies have shown that the cumulative effects of sunlight may also predispose some people to the onset of latent eye disease, usually due to heredity. However, it's not just your eyes you need to worry about. The effects of sun exposure on and around unprotected eyes can cause premature aging, sunburns, and cancer.

Doing what you can now will ensure that you and your children will have the best sight possible for years to come. Slowing down and stopping the progression of myopia with Ortho-K lenses is essential to making that future a reality. Not only will you be protecting yours or your child's eye health, but you will gain the numerous benefits of clear vision without the need for corrective lenses. Unlike other epidemics, myopia is one we can do something about.

Appendix

CANDY: **Controlling Astigmatism and Nearsightedness in Developing Youth**

David Bartels, O.D., Peter E. Wilcox, O.D.

ABSTRACT:

Background
The progressive worsening of myopia and/or astigmatic refractive errors is a serious concern for both the child and their parents. The treatment procedure known as orthokeratology has been shown to slow the rate of progression in children. This study attempted to replicate these findings.

Methods
The "No-mold" retrospective refractive data from 20 children (40 eyes) who subsequently chose orthokeratology treatment were obtained from patient records. The duration of refractive data varied from as little as 2 to as much as 82 months.

The "Molded" phase included 28 children (56 eyes). Baseline data included refraction, Simulated K (Sim K) and topographic maps. They were fit with Wave custom designed orthokeratology mold lenses. Treatment duration was 7 to 57 months.

The "Unmolded" phase involved discontinuing orthokeratology treatment until flat Sim K returned to within 1D of pre-treatment or 14 days.

Results
The mean change in spherical equivalent refractive error (SEQ) during the No-mold phase was -.37D per year. The mean change in SEQ during the Molded/Unmolded phase was -.03 D per year.

Conclusions

Orthokeratology treatment does slow the progression of myopia in children.

INTRODUCTION

The worsening of myopic and/or astigmatic refractive errors is a serious concern for both the affected child and their parents. Typical solutions include the use of spectacles and/or contact lenses. Neither of these choices addresses the concern surrounding progressive changes in refractive error but, in fairness to the clinician, there are few good options to present which work simply and predictably. There are many factors which are associated with these shifts in myopic refractive error such as: genetics (1, 2, 3), phoria (4, 5), near vision demands (6, 7), ethnicity (8, 9), sex (10) and younger age (11).

Options to slow the progression in refractive error are unpredictable and at times inconvenient.

Atropinization (12, 13) is one of the most successful forms of intervention but the side effects greatly outweigh the outcomes. Bifocals and progressive addition lenses have some effect (3, 14,) but they are cumbersome for youth with active lifestyles. Daytime wearing of rigid gas permeable lenses has been shown to slightly reduce the progression but at rates which are of limited value to the patient (15, 16).

An effective, predictable and reproducible method to reduce the rate of change of myopia and astigmatism is Orthokeratology (also known as Corneal Molding (CM), Corneal Reshaping, Corneal Refractive Therapy, Advanced Orthokeratology and Custom Accelerated Orthokeratology to name a few). Orthokeratology employs the nightly wearing of rigid gas permeable lenses (corneal molds) which reshape the curvatures of the cornea and provides great unaided vision during waking hours.

Several studies have demonstrated the effectiveness of orthokeratology. The Loric Study (20) followed patients over 12 months and concluded that Orthokeratology has a positive effect on slowing the progression of nearsightedness and astigmatism. The Orthokeratology and Adolescent Myopia Control study (21), a 3 year retrospective study, found that those who participated in orthokeratology had an average increase in myopia of only -0.67D over three years versus the expected -1.50D of change over the same period of time. In 2007, Gerowitz, Eiden and Davis initiated a similar FDA approved, 5 year corneal molding – myopia control study of 300 youths ages 8 through 14. The outcome is pending.

Methods

This study was designed to replicate the findings that orthokeratology slows the normal progression of myopia/astigmatism.

The study enrolled 28 youth. Seven were male and 21 were female. Age ranged from 4 to 20 years. Age at commencement of orthokeratology treatment ranged between 9 and 16 years.

Subjects' ethnicities were 27 Caucasians and 1 African-American. Subjects' pretreatment refractive error ranged from sphere of -1.00DS to -5.25DS (mean = -2.33D) and cylinder of plano to -1.00 (mean = 0.17DC). Mean SEQ was -2.25D.

No Mold Phase:

Historical refractive data were obtained from a subset of 20 subjects of the study group (40 eyes). They were established patients with active medical charts but had not yet begun orthokeratology treatment.

The rate of progression of their myopia during this phase was calculated as the difference between the SEQ at their first visit to the office and the SEQ just prior to initiating orthokeratology treatment.

Mold Phase:

This phase included all 28 youth (56 eyes). Refractive data prior to orthokeratology treatment were as follows: mean SEQ = -2.25D (range -1.00 to -5.50), mean sphere = -2.23D (range -1.00 to -5.25), mean cylinder = 0.17DC (range plano to -1.00).

Upon choosing orthokeratology, baseline data were collected which included a noncycloplegic refraction, topography (Scout-Eyequip), intraocular pressure and age of parents' onset of myopia/astigmatism.

The corneal molding lenses were custom designed using the captured topography maps and Wave Software System.

The dispensing visit consisted of educating the patient on the wear, insertion and removal processes and care of the lenses. A variety of care regimens were prescribed based on clinical judgment. These included Optimum and Boston cleaning and rewetting systems, Sauflon peroxide system, Allergan rewetting products and lens cleaning sponges. Following the training, unaided vision was measured. Then the patient was allowed to recline, closing their eyes for 30 minutes.

Immediately upon opening their eyes, acuities were measured and the fit was assessed with white light and NaFl. The molds were removed and topographies and unaided acuities were measured.

Though all patients initially wore their molds every night, the lens wearing schedule eventually varied among the 28 subjects: Seven wore the lenses every night, 18 wore them every second night and 3 wore then every third night. This schedule was determined by the patient and their desired endpoint acuity.

Follow up visits included one-week, one-month, three months and six months as determined by the investigators. On rare occasion, a mold lens was changed to improve fit or post wear acuity.

The treatment was considered successful if at the 3 month visit, the patient was "20/happy", topography was homogenous and no corneal pathology was observed. The duration of orthokeratology treatment varied per subject ranging from 7 to 57 months.

Unmold Phase:

Given the clinical nature of this study and inconvenience to the patient, whenever possible, an effort was made to correlate discontinuing lens wear with any unscheduled mold lens replacement (lost or broken). Otherwise, patients complied with the request to unmold.

Lens wear was discontinued and unmolding was considered complete when a subject's flat Simulated-K returned to within 1.00D of their Sim K prior to molding or 14 days had elapsed since discontinuing lens wear. During the unmolding process, noncycloplegic refractions were performed at 3 to 7 day intervals until reversal was complete.

The rate of progression of myopia for the molded patients was calculated as the difference between the SEQ just prior to molding and the SEQ after unmolding was complete.

Results

Results for all phases are presented in Figure 1. Figure 1 superimposes both the No Mold and Molded/Unmolded phase data. The X axis represents the duration of the phases in months.

No Mold Phase:

This phase included the subset of 20 established patients (40 eyes). The mean change in SEQ showed a progression of -0.37D per year. This is represented in Figure 1 by the blue data diamonds and blue trend line.

Unmold Phase:

This phase included all 28 subjects (56 eyes).

The reversal requirement was achieved by 27 of 28 subjects within two weeks (within 1D of pretreatment Sims K). In fact 44 of 54 eyes were within .5D of Sim K and 49 of 54 eyes were within .75D of original Sim K. Only 1 subject failed and was excluded from the study.

During the mold to unmold phase, the mean SEQ progression rate was only -0.03D per year. This is represented in Figure 1 by the magenta data squares and magenta trend line. Some data points are superimposed due to duplicate results on some patients. Progression rates were calculated from the raw data, not the displayed graph.

Figure 1. Myopic Progression during No Mold and Unmolded after Molding Phases

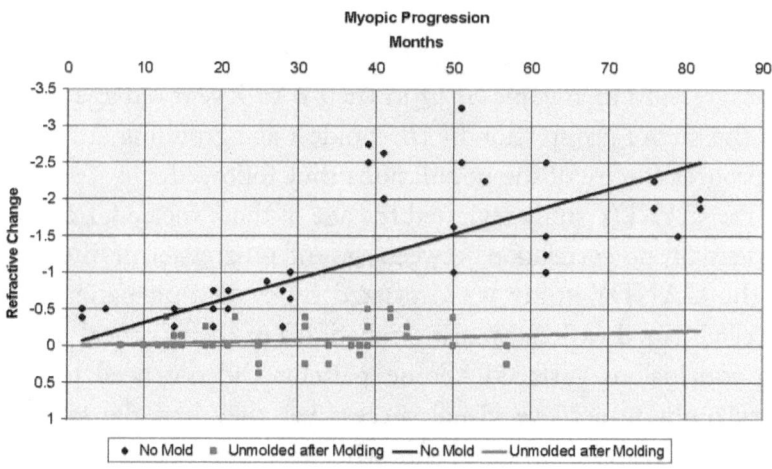

Conclusions

The CANDY study demonstrated that Orthokeratology does both significantly reduce and even stop the rate of change of nearsightedness and astigmatism in developing youth (ages 9-18). This effect was independent of the age of initiation of orthokeratology and the premolding refractive error.

This reduction in the rate of change occurs for youth in all the familial risk groups (neither, one or both parents myopic by age 18).

The IOP had no effect on myopic progression.

Discussion

The CANDY study attempted to determine if orthokeratology halted refractive error change or simply masks the change due to the molding of the corneal surface. By unmolding the treatment and allowing the Sim K's to return to baseline levels, we believe some progress has been made to answer this question. The CANDY subjects had an average **premolding** progression in their SEQ of -0.37D per year. This rate of progression in myopic children is coincident with published literature (11). These subjects' SEQ was essentially halted during the duration of their molding to an impressive mean rate of -.03D per year after being unmolded.

There is some concern that the 2 week duration of the reversal phase was insufficient despite the fact that the Sim Ks of 49 of the 54 subjects were within .75D of their baseline Sim K's. This issue should be the basis for further study. Data obtained from trials using longer reversal periods would provide more complete data.

Though Hyman, Marsh-Tootle et.al (COMET 2005) showed that there is a greater progression in myopic SEQ in their 6 to 7 year old age group and a slowing in the rate of progression by their oldest age grouping (10 to 11 years), there was progression in all the populations they followed.

When the CANDY study reviewed the age of those molded, from 9 years to 18 years, essentially no correlation between age and progression of SEQ was found.

Since the CANDY study was initiated by evaluating patients who had previously established various wearing schedules of their corneal molds, other interesting conclusions surfaced. Some patients did not need to wear their molds every night to achieve visual success yet they had the same myopia/astigmatism stabilization. The patients who were best suited to sleep in their

molds only every second to third night were those with lower refractive errors and steeper Sim K's. For this reason the authors submit that there is a greater incentive to mold the younger eye at lower refractive errors. Clinicians should present to the higher risk/lower SEQ patients and their family that:
1. orthokeratology when done in the early stages of myopia is more cost effective,
2. because their SEQ is low, it allows the child to wear the lenses every other night
3. it is more acceptable for a younger patient to experience any partial unmolding during the alternate days when the lenses were not worn
4. it is better to stop axial elongation when the eye is still shorter, reducing the risk of retinal detachment.

The population of eligible patients in this study was significantly skewed toward a white population (27 White, 1 Black, 0 Hispanic and 0 Asians). As it has been shown that there is a greater incidence of and progression of SEQ in the Asian populations (19), a similar study within a primarily Asian population would be even more powerful.

The CANDY study was designed to investigate if orthokeratology slows the progression of myopia (with or without astigmatism). The study was not designed to investigate how specifically designed corneal molds affect the eye/vision. Additionally, the goal of each patient was to have good vision (with and without the molds), good fit and good comfort; hence, liberal boundaries were granted on the complicated designs of the reverse geometry lenses. All designs were similar in they were tied to the global goals of success. An evaluation of the various designs does reveal more similarities than differences among the molds.

Despite the repeatable results of 'myopia control' by orthokeratology, some caution should be exercised in promoting this as a predictable way to halt the refractive error changes. Not all studies have found such consistent reduction in refractive error progression (Reim 2003). One of the limitations of this study is size of population. Larger, well controlled trials are needed to further validate the findings of this and other orthokeratology studies.

The investigators continue to monitor all those in the Candy study and are expanding their centers while broadening the data base. Additional variables which may be monitored are central corneal epithelial thicknesses and total central corneal thickness and axial length. They look forward to presenting their future findings.

About the authors:

Dr. Peter E. Wilcox is in solo private practice in Hayes, Virginia. He received his OD from UAB and attended a Residency at PCO.

Dr. David Bartels is in group practice in Buffalo, NY. He received his OD at ICO.

The authors would like to extend their gratitude to Caroline Guerrero Cauchi, O.D., F.O.A.A. and Richard Anderson, O.D., F.O.A.A. for their editorial assistance in preparing this article.

On a personal note, being one of the investigators and the father of two of the subjects, I am pleasantly surprised at the outcome of the study. My daughter and son both mold every 72 hours. They have been threatened with myopic progression if they don't mold more often, only to fall on deaf ears. I don't know the correct number of nights needed to hold the progression back but both my children are doing fine. Corneal Molding has become the norm in my family and it is very gratifying to observe no change in my children's vision over many years. David Bartels OD.

About the Authors

Dr. Mark J. Page, O.D.
Optometrist/Orthokeratologist

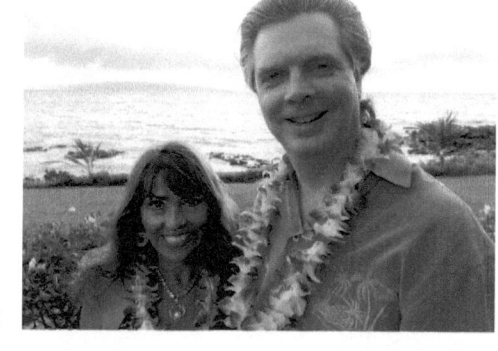

Website: www.ArizonasVision.com
Email: service@arizonasvision.com
Phone: 480-706-EYES (3937)

Dr. Page has been an Optometrist for more than twenty-five years. He has devoted his career to finding a better way. His grandmother was blind for the last five years of her life, and after he became a doctor, his father went blind in one eye. One of his older brothers had his retina tear in two places. Dr. Page is passionate about protecting his family's and his patients' eyes for a lifetime of good vision. He and his wife Gina are the proud parents of five rescue dogs and one rescue cat, and they all get along amazingly well. Dr. Page graduated from the New England College of Optometry in Boston MA.

A member of the American Optometric Association, he is also a member of the Orthokeratology Academy of America and a member of the Beta Sigma Kappa honor society. He also belongs to the Arizona Optometric Association. He has been voted as one of America's Top Optometrists. His practice, Arizona's Vision, is consistently voted as the Best of Ahwatukee. He has also been voted as Phoenix's Best Optometrist and one of Phoenix's Best Businesses. He has also appeared on ABC 15 News, Fox 10 News, and Arizona Channel 7. He has been published in the *Arizona Republic* and the *Ahwatukee Foothills News*. He has also been a part of the Orthokeratology Boot Camp at Vision By Design. He co-authored *Get Published And Grow Your Business*, which became an Amazon Best Seller. He has appeared on KFNX Radio and *Leading Experts* TV Show. He also served as an FDA clinical Investigator for contact lenses.

He enjoys playing golf with his dad and brothers, skiing with his friends, traveling to family events, reading and spending time in Maui with his wife. He started Arizona's Vision in 1994.

Dr. David M. Roth, O.D.
Optometrist/Orthokeratologist

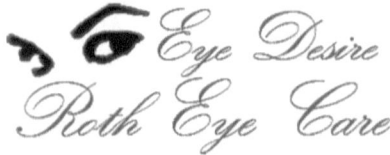
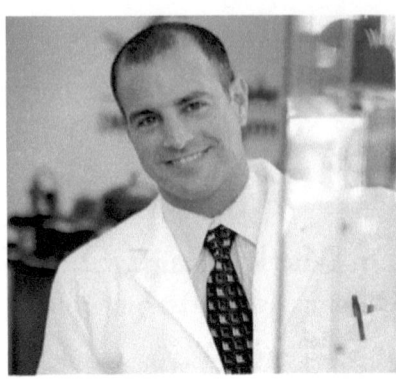

EYE DESIRE (MIAMI BEACH)
Website: www.EyeDesire.com
Phone. 305-673-1211
Fax. 305-532-7684

ROTH EYE CARE (DOWNTOWN MIAMI)
Website: www.RothEyeCare.com
Phone. 305-371-2020
Fax. 305-374-2123

Dr. David Roth is a graduate of the Illinois College of Optometry and has been in private practice for over twenty years. He is a board-certified optometric physician, as well as a certified orthokeratologist.

He is also a refractive surgery consultant for the TLC Laser Center and the Millennium Laser Center.

Part of his commitment to his patients is ongoing professional education. He is a member of the Dade County Optometric Association, the Florida Optometric Association, the Southeastern Optometric Association, the American Optometric Association, the National Educational Research Foundation, the Miami Beach Chamber of Commerce, the American Academy of Orthokeratology, VOSH International, and Young Founders of Mt. Sinai Hospital.

Optometry has been a tradition in the Roth family for three generations, and Dr. David Roth began his career working in his father's vision clinic. In 2002, he opened his own clinic and specializes in emergency eye care procedures, the diagnosis and treatment of ocular diseases, and orthokeratology.

Dr. David Roth is married, with two children. He enjoys traveling, many outdoor activities such as boating and skiing, but mostly he enjoys spending time with his family.

Dr. David P. Bartels, O.D., FIOA
Optometrist/Orthokeratologist

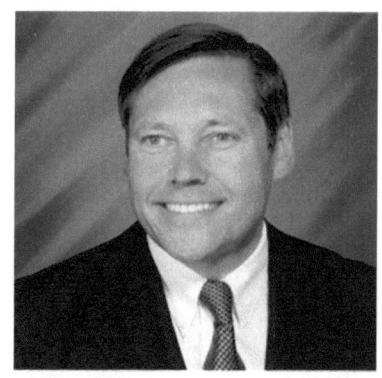

Website: www.BartelsVisionCare.com
Email: visioncare@roadrunner.com
Phone: 716-693-4606
Fax: 716-693-7329

Dr. Bartels has co-authored, published, trained, and lectured on the subject of Orthokeratogy and Scleral contacts. A graduate of the Illinois College of Optometry, AOA member, and a Fellow of the International Academy of Orthokeratogy, he practices in Buffalo, New York and is the owner of Vision Care Center, as well as a partner in Clarence Eye Care. After practicing Orthokeratogy for more than fifteen years, Dr. Bartels has developed an extensive knowledge of designing and fitting.

Dr. Michael S. Murphy, O.D.
Optometrist/Orthokeratologist

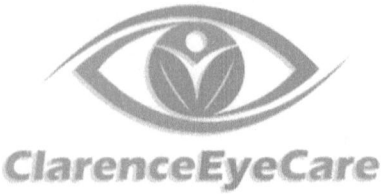

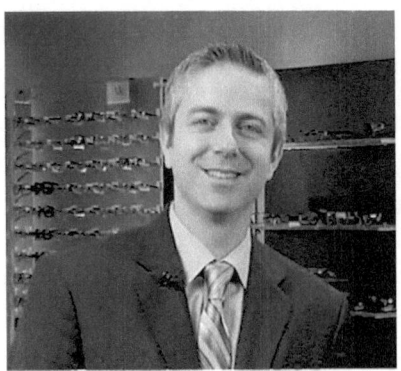

Website: www.ClarenceEyeCare.com
Email: info@clarenceeyecare.com
Phone: 716-668-2020
Fax: 716-204-8639

Michael S. Murphy, OD, earned his Bachelor of Arts from Canisius College in Buffalo, NY. He then went on to earn another Bachelor of Science in Visual Science and his Doctorate in Optometry from the Pennsylvania College of Optometry in Philadelphia, PA. He was elected vice president of his optometry class and graduated with clinical honors in primary care, ocular disease, and low vision. He currently is the vice president of his Western New York Optometric Society.

Dr. Murphy completed externships in several different modes of practice. He studied at Capital Eye Consultants in Fairfax, VA. This was a referral center for some of the most challenging eye disease patients in the Washington, DC area. It was there that he gained an understanding of ocular disease and treatment under the tutelage of Dr. John C. Baldinger and Dr. James E. Powers. Here he participated in comprehensive eye examinations, emergency eye care, cataract evaluations, glaucoma consultations, and Lasik pre- and post-operative visits. Dr. Murphy completed an externship at the Veteran's Administration Newington-Medical Center in Newington, CT, where he gained valuable experience in diagnosing eye disease pertaining to overall systemic health. He then joined a private practice in Easton, PA with Dr. John Boscia, where he gained vast knowledge in primary care and fitting of all types of contact lenses. Finally, he did a Pediatric and Low Vision rotation at The Eye Institute in Philadelphia, PA.

Today, Dr. Murphy co-owns and operates his own practice, Clarence Eye Care, with his partner Dr. David Bartels. He performs comprehensive eye examinations, with special emphasis on eye health. Dr. Murphy diagnoses diabetic eye disease, glaucoma, cataracts and other ocular pathology. He also has a special interest in contact lenses, especially orthokeratology and keratoconus. Dr. Murphy fits a wide variety of lenses, and takes interest in "hard to fit" contacts.

Dr. Murphy also continues to work for one of the busiest ophthalmology practices in Western New York, namely Fichte Endl and Elmer Eyecare. He has practiced here since graduating in spring of 2000. Here, he works closely with four ophthalmologists and four other optometrists in virtually every aspect of eye care including glaucoma and macular degeneration to Lasik and Raindrop technology.

It has also been exciting for him to bring a unique device to the optometric community. Dr. Murphy co-invented the TigerChart in 2010. It is a digital near chart that enhances the patient's experience when they are getting their eyes examined for their near-vision prescription. As part of the large ophthalmology practice, he has also had the privilege to be a co-investigator in several clinical studies including Ocular Therapeutix, ISTA Pharmaceuticals, and an Alcon Dry Eye study. He is currently an active member of the speaker alliance with Alcon giving talks to colleagues regarding the newest innovations in soft contact lens technology.

In his spare moments, Dr. Murphy likes to spend quality time with his wife Jocelyn (also an optometrist) and their two children, Jacob and Alexandria. He also enjoys biking, volleyball, camping, and attending local sporting events.

Dr. Stuart Grant, O.D.
Optometrist/Orthokeratologist

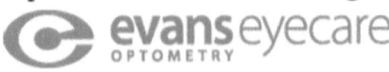

Website: www.EvansEyeCare.com
Email: info@evanseyecare.com
Phone: 760-674-8806

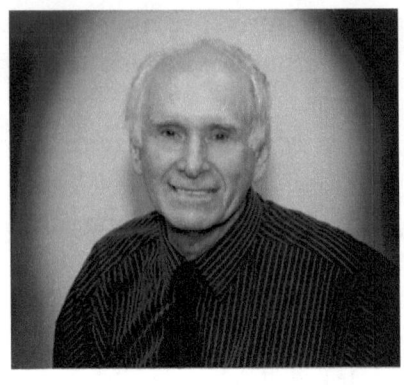

One of the founders of orthokeratology, Dr. Stuart Grant has dedicated the last six decades of his career to developing methods and technologies to stop the progression of myopia. When he is not conducting research and developing new presbyopia reverse corneal reshaping techniques, he continues to see patients at his clinic in Palm Desert, California, and specializes in complex cases, such as irregular corneas, post-surgery complications, and keratoconus (corneal) transplants.

Dr. Kevin Reeder, O.D.
Optometrist/Orthokeratologist

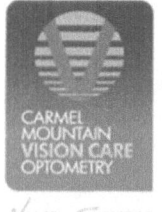
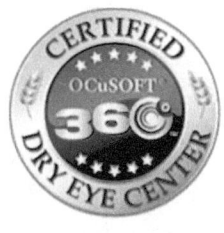
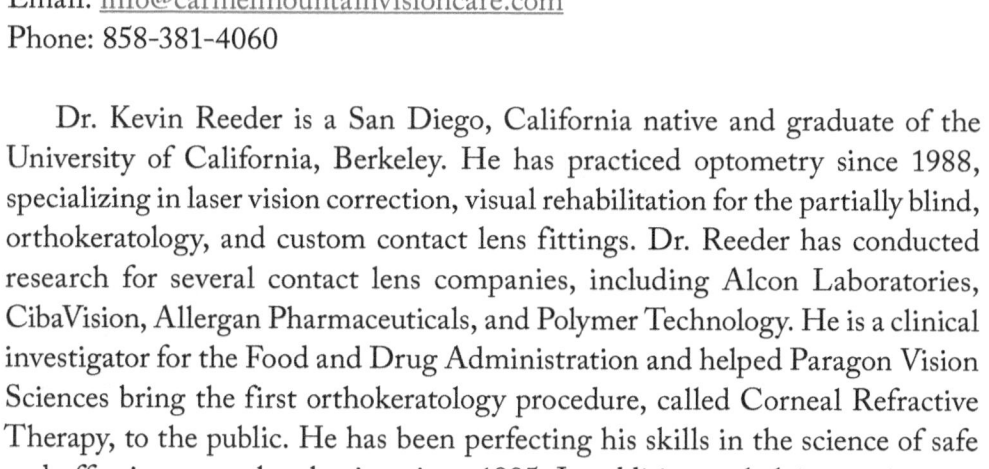

Website: CarmelMountainVisionCare.com
Email: info@carmelmountainvisioncare.com
Phone: 858-381-4060

    Dr. Kevin Reeder is a San Diego, California native and graduate of the University of California, Berkeley. He has practiced optometry since 1988, specializing in laser vision correction, visual rehabilitation for the partially blind, orthokeratology, and custom contact lens fittings. Dr. Reeder has conducted research for several contact lens companies, including Alcon Laboratories, CibaVision, Allergan Pharmaceuticals, and Polymer Technology. He is a clinical investigator for the Food and Drug Administration and helped Paragon Vision Sciences bring the first orthokeratology procedure, called Corneal Refractive Therapy, to the public. He has been perfecting his skills in the science of safe and effective corneal reshaping since 1995. In addition to helping patients at his clinic in San Diego, Dr. Reeder also provides charitable eye-care procedures through Lions In Sight.

    He lives with his wife and two children, and enjoys music and tennis.

Dr. Earl Sandler, O.D.
Optometrist/Orthokeratologist

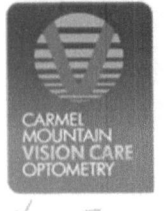
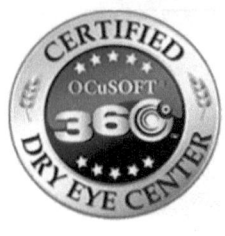
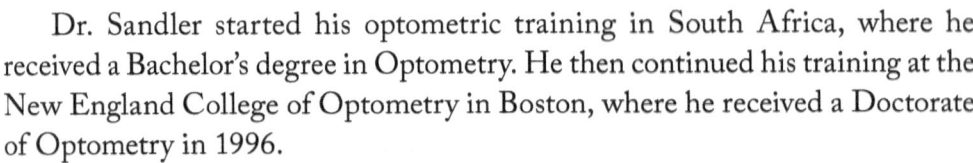

Website: CarmelMountainVisionCare.com
Email: info@carmelmountainvisioncare.com
Phone: 858-381-4060

Dr. Sandler started his optometric training in South Africa, where he received a Bachelor's degree in Optometry. He then continued his training at the New England College of Optometry in Boston, where he received a Doctorate of Optometry in 1996.

Dr. Sandler's areas of interest include specialty contact lenses and Laser Vision Correction. Dr. Sandler has been a clinical investigator and has performed research for several contact lens companies. His passion and dedication for his profession as well as his sincere attitude and caring nature enable him to provide his patients with complete and comprehensive care.

Married with two children, Dr. Sandler loves spending time with his family and also enjoys playing soccer.

Dr. Dale Tosland, O.D.
Optometrist/Orthokeratologist

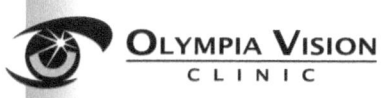

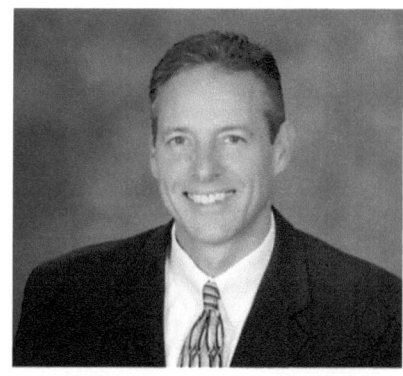

Website: OlympiaVisionClinic.com
Email: dalet@olympiavision.com
Phone: 858-381-4060

Dr. Dale L. Tosland received his Bachelor of Science degree at Pacific University in Oregon. In 1983, he earned his Doctor of Optometry degree from the Pacific University College of Optometry. Dr. Tosland completed his externship training at the Tripler Army Hospital in Honolulu, Hawaii. While in college, he served as the vice president of the Phi Beta Kappa honors fraternity. He is a member of the American Optometric Association, the Optometric Physicians of Washington, and a former president of the Olympic Society of Optometric Physicians.

His professional focus is on primary patient care, contact lenses, glaucoma, macular degeneration, diabetic eye disease, and refractive surgery. Dr. Tosland specializes in bifocal contact lenses, correction for astigmatism, and Corneal Refractive Therapy (CRT - nightwear lenses for the correction of myopia without surgery). He is a former president of the Olympia Lions Club, where he has also served as a board member. He lives in Olympia with his wife and two sons.

www.ingramcontent.com/pod-product-compliance
Lightning Source LLC
Chambersburg PA
CBHW021152080526
44588CB00008B/301